GALVESTON DIET COOKBOOK FOR BEGINNERS

2000 Days Of Recipes: Indulge In Delicious Healthy Dishes To Kick Start Your Wellness Journey. Eat Well, Feel Great With A 31-Days Meal Plan

I0781594

Wesley Hudson

Table of Contents

COPYRIGHT © 2023

CHAPTER ONE

Introduction to the Galveston Diet

The Galveston Diet is a nutritional approach developed by Dr. Mary Claire Haver, a board-certified OB-GYN, to address the specific health concerns of women in perimenopause and menopause. It focuses on balancing hormones, managing insulin resistance, and promoting overall well-being through a combination of dietary changes, intermittent fasting, and lifestyle modifications. This diet aims to alleviate symptoms commonly associated with hormonal fluctuations, such as weight gain, fatigue, mood swings, and brain fog, by optimizing nutrition and supporting metabolic health.

Understanding the Galveston Diet Philosophy

At the core of the Galveston Diet philosophy is the recognition of the unique physiological changes that occur in women as they transition through perimenopause and menopause. During this stage of life, hormonal imbalances, particularly fluctuations in estrogen and progesterone levels, can disrupt metabolism, leading to weight gain, insulin resistance, and increased risk of chronic diseases such as diabetes and cardiovascular disease.

The Galveston Diet addresses these issues by focusing on foods that support hormonal balance, stabilize blood sugar levels, and reduce inflammation. It emphasizes the importance of consuming nutrient-dense whole foods while minimizing processed foods, sugars, and refined carbohydrates. By adopting a diet rich in lean proteins, healthy fats, fiber, and phytonutrients, women can optimize their metabolism, improve insulin sensitivity, and enhance overall health and well-being.

Additionally, the Galveston Diet incorporates intermittent fasting as a tool to promote metabolic flexibility and fat loss. Intermittent fasting involves cycling between periods of eating and fasting, which can help regulate blood sugar levels, reduce insulin resistance, and promote autophagy, the body's natural process of cellular repair and regeneration.

Furthermore, the Galveston Diet emphasizes the importance of lifestyle factors such as stress management, adequate sleep, and regular physical activity in supporting hormonal balance and metabolic health. By addressing these underlying factors, women can optimize their body's ability to burn fat, maintain muscle mass, and sustain long-term weight loss success.

Overall, the Galveston Diet philosophy is rooted in a holistic approach to health and wellness, recognizing the interconnectedness of diet, hormones, and lifestyle factors in achieving optimal metabolic health and vitality during perimenopause and menopause.

Benefits of the Galveston Diet

The Galveston Diet offers a wide range of potential benefits for women in perimenopause and menopause, as well as those seeking to improve their metabolic health and overall well-being. Some of the key benefits of the Galveston Diet include:

1. Hormonal Balance: By focusing on nutrient-dense whole foods and minimizing processed foods and sugars, the Galveston Diet can help support hormonal balance by providing essential nutrients needed for hormone production and metabolism. This can help alleviate symptoms such as hot flashes, night sweats, mood swings, and fatigue associated with hormonal fluctuations during perimenopause and menopause.

2. Weight Loss: The Galveston Diet emphasizes the importance of protein-rich foods, healthy fats, and fiber to promote satiety, stabilize blood sugar levels, and enhance fat burning. By adopting a balanced and nutritious diet, women can effectively manage their weight and body composition, leading to improvements in overall health and self-confidence.

3. Improved Insulin Sensitivity: By minimizing refined carbohydrates and sugars and incorporating intermittent fasting, the Galveston Diet can help improve insulin sensitivity and reduce the risk of insulin resistance and type 2 diabetes. This can lead to better blood sugar control, lower insulin levels, and reduced inflammation, all of which are important for metabolic health and disease prevention.

4. Enhanced Energy and Mental Clarity: The Galveston Diet provides a steady source of energy by focusing on nutrient-dense whole foods and minimizing fluctuations in blood sugar levels. This can help alleviate fatigue, brain fog, and mood swings commonly experienced during perimenopause and menopause, allowing women to feel more energized, focused, and mentally sharp throughout the day.

5. Cardiovascular Health: The Galveston Diet promotes heart-healthy eating habits by emphasizing the consumption of lean proteins, healthy fats, and fiber-rich foods while minimizing processed foods and trans fats. This can help lower cholesterol levels, reduce inflammation, and improve other risk factors associated with cardiovascular disease, such as high blood pressure and obesity.

6. Longevity and Aging: By supporting metabolic health, hormonal balance, and cellular repair mechanisms, the Galveston Diet may contribute to longevity and healthy aging. Intermittent fasting, in particular, has been shown to promote autophagy, the body's natural process of cellular cleanup and renewal, which may help slow down the aging process and reduce the risk of age-related diseases.

Overall, the Galveston Diet offers a comprehensive approach to health and wellness that addresses the unique needs of women in perimenopause and menopause, while also providing numerous benefits for metabolic health, weight management, and overall vitality.

Getting Started: Essential Tools and Ingredients

Getting started with the Galveston Diet requires some essential tools and ingredients to set yourself up for success. Here are some key components to consider:

1. **Nutrient-Dense Foods**: The foundation of the Galveston Diet is built on nutrient-dense whole foods such as lean proteins, healthy fats, fruits, vegetables, and whole grains. Stock your pantry and refrigerator with a variety of fresh, minimally processed ingredients to create balanced and satisfying meals.

2. **Protein Sources**: Incorporate a variety of protein sources into your diet, including poultry, fish, eggs, tofu, legumes, and dairy products. Protein helps promote satiety, support muscle growth and repair, and stabilize blood sugar levels, making it an essential component of the Galveston Diet.

3. **Healthy Fats**: Include healthy fats in your meals from sources such as avocados, nuts, seeds, olive oil, and fatty fish. Healthy fats provide essential fatty acids, fat-soluble vitamins, and antioxidants, which are important for hormone production, brain health, and inflammation management.

4. **Fiber-Rich Foods**: Aim to include plenty of fiber-rich foods in your diet, such as fruits, vegetables, whole grains, beans, and lentils. Fiber helps promote digestive health, regulate blood sugar levels, and support weight management by promoting feelings of fullness and satiety.

5. **Low-Glycemic Carbohydrates**: Choose carbohydrates that are low on the glycemic index, such as whole grains, sweet potatoes, quinoa, and legumes, to help stabilize blood sugar levels and reduce the risk of insulin resistance. Limit refined carbohydrates and sugars, which can cause rapid spikes and crashes in blood sugar levels.

6. **Intermittent Fasting**: Consider incorporating intermittent fasting into your routine as a tool to support metabolic health and fat loss. Start with a simple fasting schedule, such as fasting for 12-16 hours overnight or incorporating one or two 24-hour fasts per week, and gradually adjust based on your individual needs and preferences.

7. **Hydration**: Stay hydrated by drinking plenty of water throughout the day. Hydration is essential for supporting metabolic processes, promoting digestion, and maintaining overall health and well-being. Aim to drink at least 8-10 glasses of water per day, and consider incorporating herbal teas, infused water, or electrolyte drinks for variety.

8. **Meal Planning and Preparation**: Take time to plan and prepare your meals ahead of time to ensure you have nutritious options readily available. Batch cooking, meal prepping, and using meal delivery services can help simplify the process and save time during busy weekdays.

9. **Mindful Eating Practices**: Practice mindful eating by paying attention to hunger and fullness cues, savoring each bite, and avoiding distractions such as screens or multitasking while eating. Mindful eating can help promote healthier food choices, improve digestion, and enhance overall satisfaction with meals.

10. **Support and Accountability**: Consider seeking support from a healthcare provider, nutritionist, or online community to help you stay motivated and accountable on your Galveston Diet journey. Surround yourself with like-minded individuals who can offer encouragement, share tips and recipes, and celebrate your successes along the way.

By incorporating these essential tools and ingredients into your lifestyle, you can embark on a successful Galveston Diet journey and experience the many benefits it has to offer for hormonal balance, metabolic health, and overall well-being. Remember to listen to your body, experiment with different foods and fasting protocols, and make adjustments as needed to find what works best for you.

CHAPTER TWO

Breakfast Recipes

Breakfast is often considered the most important meal of the day, setting the tone for your energy levels and metabolism. When following the Galveston Diet, it's essential to start your day with nutritious and satisfying meals that support hormonal balance and provide lasting energy. Here are three delicious breakfast recipes to fuel your morning and kickstart your metabolism:

Energizing Morning Smoothies

Smoothies are a convenient and delicious way to pack in essential nutrients, fiber, and antioxidants first thing in the morning. By incorporating a variety of fruits, vegetables, protein sources, and healthy fats, you can create a balanced and energizing breakfast option that will keep you feeling full and focused throughout the morning.

Ingredients:

- 1 cup leafy greens (such as spinach or kale)
- 1/2 frozen banana
- 1/2 cup frozen berries (such as strawberries, blueberries, or raspberries)
- 1/4 avocado
- 1 scoop protein powder (such as whey, pea, or collagen)

- 1 tablespoon chia seeds or flaxseeds

- 1 cup unsweetened almond milk or coconut water

Instructions:

1. In a blender, combine the leafy greens, frozen banana, frozen berries, avocado, protein powder, and chia seeds or flaxseeds.

2. Pour in the unsweetened almond milk or coconut water.

3. Blend until smooth and creamy, adding more liquid as needed to reach your desired consistency.

4. Pour into a glass and enjoy immediately as a refreshing and nourishing breakfast option.

Protein-Packed Breakfast Bowls

Breakfast bowls are a versatile and customizable option that allows you to mix and match your favorite ingredients to create a satisfying and nutritious meal. By combining protein-rich foods, healthy fats, and fiber-packed carbohydrates, you can create a balanced breakfast bowl that will keep you full and satisfied until your next meal.

Ingredients:

- 1/2 cup cooked quinoa or oats

- 1/4 cup Greek yogurt or coconut yogurt

- 1/4 cup mixed berries

- 1 tablespoon almond butter or peanut butter

- 1 tablespoon unsweetened coconut flakes

- 1 tablespoon pumpkin seeds or sunflower seeds

- Drizzle of honey or maple syrup (optional)

- Dash of cinnamon or nutmeg (optional)

Instructions:

1. In a bowl, layer the cooked quinoa or oats as the base.

2. Top with Greek yogurt or coconut yogurt.

3. Add mixed berries, almond butter or peanut butter, coconut flakes, and pumpkin seeds or sunflower seeds.

4. Drizzle with honey or maple syrup and sprinkle with cinnamon or nutmeg, if desired.

5. Mix everything together until well combined, and enjoy your protein-packed breakfast bowl for a satisfying and nutritious start to your day.

Flavorful Egg Variations

Eggs are a nutrient-dense and versatile ingredient that can be prepared in countless delicious ways. Whether scrambled, poached, boiled, or baked, eggs are an excellent source of high-quality protein, vitamins, and minerals, making them an ideal choice for breakfast on the Galveston Diet.

Ingredients:

- 2 eggs

- 1/4 cup diced vegetables (such as bell peppers, onions, spinach, mushrooms, or tomatoes)

- 1/4 cup shredded cheese (such as cheddar, mozzarella, or feta)

- 1 tablespoon chopped fresh herbs (such as parsley, cilantro, or basil)

- Salt and pepper to taste

- Cooking oil or butter for greasing the pan

Instructions:

1. In a bowl, whisk together the eggs until well beaten.

2. Heat a non-stick skillet over medium heat and add a small amount of cooking oil or butter to grease the pan.

3. Add the diced vegetables to the skillet and sauté until softened, about 2-3 minutes.

4. Pour the beaten eggs into the skillet, stirring gently with a spatula to scramble.

5. Once the eggs are almost set, sprinkle the shredded cheese over the top and continue cooking until melted and creamy.

6. Remove from heat and transfer the scrambled eggs to a plate.

7. Garnish with chopped fresh herbs and season with salt and pepper to taste.

8. Serve your flavorful egg variation alongside whole grain toast, sliced avocado, or a side of fresh fruit for a nutritious and satisfying breakfast option.

These breakfast recipes are designed to provide you with the energy and nutrients you need to start your day off right while following the Galveston Diet. Feel free to customize them based on your personal preferences and dietary needs, and enjoy the delicious flavors and nourishing benefits they have to offer.

CHAPTER THREE

Lunchtime Delights

Lunch is a crucial meal that refuels your body and provides the necessary energy to sustain you throughout the day. When following the Galveston Diet, it's important to prioritize nutrient-dense meals that support hormonal balance and promote overall well-being. Here are three satisfying and delicious lunchtime options to enjoy:

Fresh and Vibrant Salads

Salads are a versatile and nutritious option for lunch, allowing you to incorporate a variety of fresh vegetables, lean proteins, healthy fats, and flavorful dressings. By combining different textures and flavors, you can create a satisfying and vibrant salad that will keep you feeling full and energized throughout the afternoon.

Ingredients:

- Mixed greens (such as spinach, arugula, kale, or romaine lettuce)

- Assorted vegetables (such as cucumbers, tomatoes, bell peppers, carrots, and radishes)

- Protein source (such as grilled chicken, salmon, tofu, chickpeas, or hard-boiled eggs)

- Healthy fats (such as avocado slices, nuts, seeds, or feta cheese)

- Dressing (such as olive oil and balsamic vinegar, lemon tahini, or honey mustard)

Instructions:

1. In a large bowl, combine the mixed greens and assorted vegetables of your choice.

2. Add your protein source and healthy fats to the salad, arranging them evenly on top.

3. Drizzle with your favorite dressing, tossing gently to coat all the ingredients.

4. Optional: garnish with fresh herbs, crumbled cheese, or additional toppings for added flavor and texture.

5. Serve your fresh and vibrant salad as a satisfying and nutritious lunch option that will keep you feeling full and satisfied throughout the afternoon.

Hearty Soups and Stews

Soups and stews are comforting and nourishing options for lunch, especially during the colder months. They are a great way to pack in plenty of vegetables, lean proteins, and healthy fats, making them a balanced and satisfying meal choice on the Galveston Diet.

Ingredients:

- Assorted vegetables (such as onions, carrots, celery, bell peppers, and zucchini)

- Protein source (such as chicken breast, turkey sausage, lean beef, or tofu)

- Low-sodium broth or stock (such as chicken, vegetable, or beef)

- Whole grains (such as quinoa, brown rice, or barley)

- Herbs and spices (such as garlic, thyme, rosemary, and paprika)

- Healthy fats (such as olive oil, avocado, or coconut milk)

Instructions:

1. In a large pot or Dutch oven, heat a small amount of olive oil over medium heat.

2. Add the chopped onions, carrots, celery, and bell peppers to the pot, sautéing until softened, about 5-7 minutes.

3. Add your protein source to the pot, cooking until browned and cooked through.

4. Pour in the low-sodium broth or stock, along with any additional vegetables, whole grains, herbs, and spices.

5. Bring the soup to a boil, then reduce the heat and let it simmer for 20-30 minutes, until the flavors have melded together and the vegetables are tender.

6. Taste and adjust the seasoning as needed, adding salt, pepper, or additional herbs and spices to taste.

7. Serve your hearty soup or stew hot, garnished with fresh herbs or a dollop of Greek yogurt, for a comforting and satisfying lunch option that will keep you warm and full throughout the afternoon.

Savory Sandwiches and Wraps

Sandwiches and wraps are convenient and portable options for lunch, allowing you to pack in a variety of flavors and textures into a handheld meal. By choosing whole grain bread or wraps and filling them with lean proteins, plenty of vegetables, and flavorful spreads, you can create a balanced and satisfying lunch option that will keep you fueled and satisfied until dinner.

Ingredients:

- Whole grain bread or wrap

- Protein source (such as turkey breast, grilled chicken, tuna salad, or tofu)

- Assorted vegetables (such as lettuce, spinach, tomatoes, cucumbers, and avocado)

- Healthy fats (such as hummus, guacamole, or tahini)

- Flavorful spreads (such as mustard, pesto, or Greek yogurt dressing)

Instructions:

1. Lay out your whole grain bread or wrap on a clean surface.

2. Spread your favorite flavorful spread evenly over the bread or wrap, leaving a small border around the edges.

3. Layer your protein source, assorted vegetables, and healthy fats on top of the spread, arranging them evenly across the surface.

4. Optional: sprinkle with herbs, spices, or additional toppings for added flavor and texture.

5. Carefully roll up the sandwich or wrap, folding in the sides as you go, until all the ingredients are enclosed.

6. Slice the sandwich or wrap in half, if desired, and serve immediately as a convenient and satisfying lunch option that can be enjoyed at home or on the go.

These lunchtime delights offer a variety of delicious and nutritious options to enjoy while following the Galveston Diet. Whether you prefer fresh and vibrant salads, hearty soups and stews, or savory sandwiches and wraps, there's something for everyone to enjoy that will keep you feeling full and energized throughout the day. Experiment with different ingredients, flavors, and textures to create your own customized meals that support your health and well-being.

CHAPTER FOUR

Snack Attack

Snacking can be a crucial part of maintaining energy levels and preventing overeating during meals. However, it's important to choose snacks that are nutritious and satisfying, especially when following the Galveston Diet. Here are three categories of snack ideas that are not only delicious but also align with the principles of the Galveston Diet:

Nutritious Snack Ideas for Anytime

When it comes to snacks, opting for nutrient-dense options can help keep hunger at bay and provide essential vitamins and minerals to support overall health. Here are some nutritious snack ideas that you can enjoy anytime:

- **Greek Yogurt Parfait**: Layer Greek yogurt with fresh berries, nuts, and a drizzle of honey or maple syrup for a protein-rich and satisfying snack.

- **Apple Slices with Almond Butter**: Slice up an apple and pair it with a tablespoon of almond butter for a delicious combination of fiber, healthy fats, and natural sweetness.

- **Vegetable Sticks with Hummus**: Cut up carrots, cucumber, bell peppers, and celery sticks and serve them with a side of hummus for a crunchy and satisfying snack packed with vitamins, minerals, and fiber.

- **Hard-Boiled Eggs**: Hard-boiled eggs are a convenient and portable snack option that provides high-quality protein and essential nutrients to keep you feeling full and energized.

- **Mixed Nuts and Seeds**: Create your own trail mix by combining a variety of nuts and seeds, such as almonds, walnuts, pumpkin seeds, and sunflower seeds, for a crunchy and nutrient-rich snack.

Guilt-Free Dips and Spreads

Dips and spreads can add flavor and texture to your snacks while providing essential nutrients and healthy fats. Here are some guilt-free dip and spread ideas to enjoy with your favorite snacks:

- **Guacamole**: Mash ripe avocados with lime juice, minced garlic, diced tomatoes, chopped cilantro, and a pinch of salt for a creamy and flavorful dip that pairs well with vegetable sticks or whole grain crackers.

- **Greek Yogurt Dip**: Mix Greek yogurt with lemon zest, minced garlic, chopped fresh dill, and a dash of black pepper for a tangy and protein-rich dip that goes perfectly with raw vegetables or pita chips.

- **Hummus**: Blend chickpeas with tahini, lemon juice, garlic, olive oil, and a sprinkle of paprika for a smooth and creamy hummus that is packed with fiber, protein, and healthy fats.

- **Nut Butter**: Spread almond butter, peanut butter, or cashew butter on whole grain crackers, rice cakes, or apple slices for a satisfying and nutritious snack that provides a good balance of protein, carbohydrates, and healthy fats.

- **Tzatziki**: Combine Greek yogurt with grated cucumber, minced garlic, chopped fresh mint, lemon juice, and a pinch of salt for a refreshing and cooling dip that pairs well with raw vegetables or whole grain pita bread.

Crunchy and Satisfying Trail Mixes

Trail mixes are a convenient and portable snack option that combines a variety of nuts, seeds, dried fruits, and other tasty ingredients. Here are some crunchy and satisfying trail mix ideas to enjoy on the go:

- **Classic Trail Mix**: Combine almonds, walnuts, cashews, pumpkin seeds, and dried cranberries for a classic trail mix that offers a good balance of protein, healthy fats, and carbohydrates.

- **Tropical Trail Mix**: Mix together macadamia nuts, coconut flakes, dried pineapple, banana chips, and dark chocolate chunks for a tropical-inspired trail mix that is sweet, crunchy, and satisfying.

- **Spicy Trail Mix**: Toss together roasted chickpeas, almonds, cashews, pumpkin seeds, and a sprinkle of chili powder, cayenne pepper, and smoked paprika for a spicy and savory trail mix that packs a punch.

- **Chocolate Lover's Trail Mix**: Combine dark chocolate chips, almonds, cashews, dried cherries, and coconut flakes for a decadent and indulgent trail mix that satisfies your sweet tooth while providing a boost of energy and nutrients.

- **Superfood Trail Mix**: Mix together goji berries, goldenberries, cacao nibs, pumpkin seeds, and hemp seeds for a nutrient-rich trail mix that is packed with antioxidants, vitamins, and minerals.

These snack ideas are not only delicious and satisfying but also align with the principles of the Galveston Diet by providing nutrient-dense options that support hormonal balance and overall well-being. Whether you're craving something sweet, savory, or crunchy, there's a snack option for every taste preference and dietary need. Experiment with different ingredients and flavor combinations to create your own customized snacks that keep you feeling full, energized, and satisfied throughout the day.

CHAPTER FIVE

Dinner Creations

Dinner is a time to unwind and nourish your body with a satisfying and balanced meal. When following the Galveston Diet, it's important to choose dinner options that are not only delicious but also support hormonal balance and overall health. Here are three categories of dinner creations that are sure to delight your taste buds:

Wholesome One-Pot Meals

One-pot meals are a convenient and efficient way to prepare a nutritious dinner with minimal cleanup. These wholesome dishes often combine protein, vegetables, and grains or legumes in a single pot, creating a balanced and satisfying meal that the whole family will enjoy. Here are some ideas for wholesome one-pot meals:

- **Vegetable Stir-Fry with Quinoa**: Sauté chopped vegetables such as bell peppers, broccoli, carrots, and snap peas in a wok or large skillet with garlic, ginger, and your choice of protein (tofu, chicken, shrimp, or beef). Add cooked quinoa and a splash of soy sauce or teriyaki sauce, and toss everything together until heated through and well combined.

- **Turkey and Vegetable Chili**: Brown ground turkey in a large pot or Dutch oven with onions, garlic, bell peppers, and spices such as chili powder, cumin, and paprika. Add canned tomatoes, kidney beans, black beans, and corn, along with broth or water, and let simmer until the flavors have melded together and the chili is thick and hearty.

- **Lemon Herb Chicken and Rice**: Season chicken thighs with lemon zest, garlic, thyme, rosemary, salt, and pepper, and sear them in a skillet until golden brown. Remove the chicken from the skillet and add chopped vegetables such as onions, bell peppers, and zucchini, along with uncooked rice and chicken broth. Nestle the chicken back into the skillet, cover, and let simmer until the rice is cooked and the chicken is tender.

- **Vegetarian Lentil Curry**: Sauté onions, garlic, ginger, and curry paste in a large pot or Dutch oven until fragrant. Add red lentils, diced tomatoes, coconut milk, and vegetable broth, and let simmer until the lentils are tender and the curry is thick and creamy. Serve over cooked rice or quinoa, garnished with fresh cilantro and a squeeze of lime juice.

Flavorful Fish and Seafood Dishes

Fish and seafood are excellent sources of protein, omega-3 fatty acids, and essential nutrients, making them a healthy and delicious choice for dinner. Whether grilled, baked, or sautéed, fish and seafood dishes are versatile and flavorful options that can be enjoyed in a variety of ways. Here are some ideas for flavorful fish and seafood dishes:

- **Grilled Salmon with Lemon Herb Butter**: Season salmon fillets with salt, pepper, and a squeeze of lemon juice, and grill them over medium heat until cooked through and flaky. Serve the grilled salmon with a dollop of lemon herb butter made with softened butter, chopped fresh herbs (such as dill, parsley, and chives), and lemon zest.

- **Shrimp and Vegetable Skewers**: Thread large shrimp onto skewers alternating with colorful vegetables such as cherry tomatoes, bell peppers, zucchini, and red onion. Brush the skewers with olive oil and season with salt, pepper, and your favorite herbs and spices, then grill or broil until the shrimp are pink and cooked through.

- **Baked Cod with Tomato Basil Sauce**: Season cod fillets with salt, pepper, and olive oil, and place them in a baking dish. Top the cod with a flavorful tomato basil sauce made with diced tomatoes, garlic, onions, fresh basil, and a splash of white wine or broth. Bake the cod in the oven until tender and flaky, and serve hot with a side of steamed vegetables or whole grains.

- **Crispy Coconut Shrimp with Mango Salsa**: Dip large shrimp in beaten egg, then coat them in a mixture of shredded coconut and breadcrumbs seasoned with salt, pepper, and paprika. Fry the coconut shrimp in coconut oil until golden brown and crispy, and serve them with a fresh mango salsa made with diced mango, red bell pepper, red onion, cilantro, lime juice, and jalapeño.

Comforting Casseroles and Bakes

Casseroles and bakes are comforting and satisfying dishes that are perfect for busy weeknights or when feeding a crowd. These hearty meals often combine protein, vegetables, and grains in a single dish, making them a convenient and nutritious option for dinner. Here are some ideas for comforting casseroles and bakes:

- **Chicken and Vegetable Casserole**: Layer cooked chicken breast or thighs with steamed vegetables such as broccoli, cauliflower, and carrots in a baking dish. Top the casserole with a mixture of Greek yogurt, Dijon mustard, garlic, and grated cheese, and bake in the oven until bubbly and golden brown.

- **Vegetarian Quinoa Bake**: Combine cooked quinoa with sautéed vegetables such as spinach, mushrooms, onions, and bell peppers in a baking dish. Stir in canned beans (such as black beans or chickpeas), diced tomatoes, and your favorite spices and herbs, then top with shredded cheese and bake until heated through and bubbly.

- **Beef and Sweet Potato Shepherd's Pie**: Brown lean ground beef with onions, garlic, and mixed vegetables such as peas and carrots in a skillet. Transfer the beef mixture to a baking dish and top with mashed sweet potatoes seasoned with butter, milk, and nutmeg. Bake the shepherd's pie in the oven until the sweet potatoes are golden brown and the filling is bubbling.

- **Spinach and Ricotta Stuffed Shells**: Stuff cooked pasta shells with a mixture of ricotta cheese, cooked spinach, garlic, and grated Parmesan cheese. Arrange the stuffed shells in a baking dish and cover with marinara sauce and shredded mozzarella cheese, then bake in the oven until hot and bubbly.

These dinner creations offer a variety of delicious and nutritious options to enjoy while following the Galveston Diet. Whether you prefer wholesome one-pot meals, flavorful fish and seafood dishes, or comforting casseroles and bakes, there's something for everyone to enjoy that will satisfy your taste buds and support your health and well-being. Experiment with different ingredients, flavors, and cooking techniques to create your own customized dinners that nourish your body and bring joy to your dinner table.

CHAPTER SIX
Satisfying Side Dishes

Side dishes complement main courses and add variety and nutrition to your meals. When following the Galveston Diet, it's important to choose side dishes that are not only satisfying and delicious but also support hormonal balance and overall health. Here are three categories of side dishes that are sure to enhance your meals:

Colorful Veggie Medleys

Vegetables are packed with essential vitamins, minerals, and antioxidants, making them an excellent choice for side dishes. Colorful veggie medleys combine a variety of vegetables to create a visually appealing and nutrient-rich accompaniment to your main course. Here are some ideas for colorful veggie medleys:

- **Roasted Root Vegetables**: Toss chopped root vegetables such as carrots, sweet potatoes, parsnips, and beets with olive oil, garlic, and herbs such as rosemary and thyme. Roast the vegetables in the oven until tender and caramelized, then sprinkle with sea salt and serve hot as a flavorful and colorful side dish.

- **Sautéed Green Beans with Almonds**: Sauté fresh green beans with sliced almonds, garlic, and lemon zest in a skillet until tender-crisp and bright green. Season with salt, pepper, and a squeeze of lemon juice, then transfer to a serving dish and garnish with chopped fresh parsley for a simple and vibrant side dish.

- **Stir-Fried Asian Vegetables**: Stir-fry a colorful mix of vegetables such as bell peppers, snap peas, broccoli, carrots, and cabbage in a wok with garlic, ginger, and soy sauce. Cook until the vegetables are crisp-tender and the flavors have melded together, then serve hot as a flavorful and nutritious side dish.

- **Grilled Vegetable Platter**: Grill a variety of vegetables such as zucchini, eggplant, bell peppers, mushrooms, and asparagus until tender and lightly charred. Arrange the grilled vegetables on a platter and drizzle with balsamic glaze or a squeeze of lemon juice, then sprinkle with fresh herbs such as basil or mint for a colorful and flavorful side dish.

Protein-Packed Grain Alternatives

Grains provide energy-sustaining carbohydrates and essential nutrients, but when following the Galveston Diet, it's important to choose whole grain alternatives that are rich in fiber and protein. Here are some ideas for protein-packed grain alternatives:

- **Quinoa Pilaf**: Cook quinoa in vegetable or chicken broth with diced onions, garlic, and herbs such as parsley and thyme until fluffy and tender. Fluff the cooked quinoa with a fork and stir in toasted nuts or seeds such as almonds, pistachios, or pumpkin seeds for added crunch and protein.

- **Cauliflower Rice Stir-Fry**: Pulse cauliflower florets in a food processor until they resemble rice grains, then sauté the cauliflower rice in a skillet with diced vegetables such as bell peppers, onions, and peas. Add scrambled eggs or tofu for extra protein, along with soy sauce and sesame oil for flavor.

- **Lentil Salad**: Cook lentils in vegetable or chicken broth with diced onions, garlic, and bay leaves until tender but still firm, then drain and let cool. Toss the cooked lentils with chopped vegetables such as cucumbers, tomatoes, and bell peppers, along with fresh herbs such as parsley and mint, and a simple vinaigrette made with olive oil, lemon juice, and Dijon mustard.

- **Chickpea Curry**: Sauté diced onions, garlic, and ginger in a skillet until softened, then add canned chickpeas along with diced tomatoes, coconut milk, and curry powder. Simmer the chickpea curry until thick and flavorful, then serve hot over cooked brown rice or quinoa for a protein-rich and satisfying side dish.

Homemade Sauces and Dressings

Sauces and dressings add flavor and moisture to your meals while enhancing their nutritional value. Homemade sauces and dressings allow you to control the ingredients and customize the flavor to your liking. Here are some ideas for homemade sauces and dressings:

- **Basil Pesto**: Blend fresh basil leaves with garlic, pine nuts, Parmesan cheese, and olive oil until smooth and creamy. Use basil pesto as a sauce for pasta, grilled vegetables, or baked chicken, or toss it with cooked grains or legumes for added flavor.

- **Greek Yogurt Ranch Dressing**: Mix Greek yogurt with minced garlic, chopped fresh dill, parsley, chives, and a squeeze of lemon juice. Season with salt and pepper to taste, and use Greek yogurt ranch dressing as a dip for vegetable sticks, a topping for salads, or a sauce for grilled meats or seafood.

- **Tahini Sauce**: Whisk tahini with lemon juice, minced garlic, water, and a pinch of salt until smooth and creamy. Drizzle tahini sauce over roasted vegetables, falafel, or grain bowls, or use it as a dip for pita bread or raw vegetables for a creamy and tangy flavor.

- **Balsamic Glaze**: Simmer balsamic vinegar with honey or maple syrup in a saucepan over medium heat until thick and syrupy. Use balsamic glaze as a drizzle for grilled vegetables, roasted meats, or Caprese salads, or mix it with olive oil and Dijon mustard for a tangy salad dressing.

These satisfying side dishes add flavor, nutrition, and variety to your meals while supporting the principles of the Galveston Diet. Whether you choose colorful veggie medleys, protein-packed grain alternatives, or homemade sauces and dressings, there's something for everyone to enjoy that will complement your main course and nourish your body. Experiment with different ingredients, flavors, and cooking techniques to create your own customized side dishes that enhance your meals and bring joy to your dinner table.

CHAPTER SEVEN

Decadent Desserts

Desserts are a delightful way to indulge your sweet tooth while still adhering to the principles of the Galveston Diet. By choosing wholesome ingredients and mindful portion sizes, you can enjoy decadent desserts that satisfy your cravings without compromising your health goals. Here are three categories of decadent desserts that are sure to satisfy your sweet cravings:

Indulgent Yet Healthy Treats

Indulgent yet healthy treats are a perfect way to enjoy dessert guilt-free. By using nutritious ingredients and natural sweeteners, you can create decadent desserts that nourish your body and satisfy your taste buds. Here are some ideas for indulgent yet healthy treats:

- **Avocado Chocolate Mousse**: Blend ripe avocados with cocoa powder, dates, vanilla extract, and a splash of almond milk until smooth and creamy. Chill the mixture in the refrigerator until set, then serve topped with fresh berries and chopped nuts for a rich and satisfying dessert.

- **Chia Seed Pudding**: Mix chia seeds with unsweetened almond milk, vanilla extract, and a touch of maple syrup or honey. Let the mixture sit in the refrigerator until thick and creamy, then serve layered with sliced bananas, coconut flakes, and a drizzle of almond butter for a nutritious and satisfying pudding.

- **Banana Ice Cream**: Freeze ripe bananas until firm, then blend them in a food processor until smooth and creamy. Add a splash of almond milk or coconut milk to help with blending, along with flavorings such as cocoa powder, peanut butter, or frozen berries for a creamy and indulgent ice cream alternative.

- **Nutty Energy Bites**: Combine dates, nuts, seeds, and spices such as cinnamon and nutmeg in a food processor until finely chopped and sticky. Roll the mixture into small balls, then coat them in shredded coconut, cocoa powder, or crushed nuts for a satisfying and portable snack or dessert.

Fruit-Filled Delights

Fruit-filled delights are a refreshing and naturally sweet option for dessert. By incorporating fresh or frozen fruits into your desserts, you can enjoy a burst of flavor and nutrition with every bite. Here are some ideas for fruit-filled delights:

- **Mixed Berry Crisp**: Toss mixed berries with a squeeze of lemon juice, a sprinkle of cinnamon, and a touch of maple syrup or honey. Transfer the berry mixture to a baking dish, then top with a mixture of oats, almond flour, coconut oil, and chopped nuts. Bake in the oven until the berries are bubbling and the topping is golden brown and crisp, then serve hot with a dollop of Greek yogurt or coconut whipped cream for a delicious and satisfying dessert.

- **Grilled Pineapple with Coconut Yogurt**: Slice fresh pineapple into rings and grill them until caramelized and slightly charred. Serve the grilled pineapple with a dollop of coconut yogurt and a sprinkle of toasted coconut flakes for a tropical-inspired dessert that is both refreshing and indulgent.

- **Stuffed Baked Apples**: Core apples and stuff them with a mixture of chopped nuts, dried fruit, cinnamon, and a drizzle of honey or maple syrup. Bake the stuffed apples in the oven until tender and fragrant, then serve hot with a scoop of vanilla ice cream or a dollop of whipped cream for a comforting and satisfying dessert.

- **Chocolate-Dipped Strawberries**: Dip fresh strawberries into melted dark chocolate and place them on a parchment-lined baking sheet. Chill the chocolate-dipped strawberries in the refrigerator until the chocolate is set, then serve as a simple and elegant dessert that is perfect for special occasions or everyday indulgence.

Guilt-Free Chocolate Confections

Chocolate confections are a decadent treat that can be enjoyed in moderation on the Galveston Diet. By choosing dark chocolate with a high cocoa content and incorporating it into your desserts in creative ways, you can satisfy your chocolate cravings without derailing your health goals. Here are some ideas for guilt-free chocolate confections:

- **Dark Chocolate Bark**: Melt dark chocolate and spread it in a thin layer on a parchment-lined baking sheet. Sprinkle the melted chocolate with chopped nuts, dried fruit, shredded coconut, and a pinch of sea salt, then chill in the refrigerator until set. Break the chocolate bark into pieces and serve as a satisfying and customizable dessert or snack.

- **Chocolate Avocado Brownies**: Blend ripe avocados with cocoa powder, eggs, almond flour, maple syrup or honey, vanilla extract, and a pinch of salt until smooth and creamy. Fold in chocolate chips or chopped nuts, then pour the batter into a greased baking dish and bake in the oven until set and fudgy. Let the brownies cool completely before slicing and serving for a rich and indulgent dessert.

- **Chocolate-Covered Almonds**: Melt dark chocolate and dip whole almonds into the melted chocolate until coated. Place the chocolate-covered almonds on a parchment-lined baking sheet and chill in the refrigerator until the chocolate is set, then serve as a crunchy and satisfying snack or dessert.

- **Chocolate Coconut Truffles**: Mix melted dark chocolate with coconut cream, shredded coconut, and a splash of vanilla extract until smooth and creamy. Roll the chocolate coconut mixture into small balls, then coat them in cocoa powder, chopped nuts, or shredded coconut for a decadent and irresistible treat.

These decadent desserts offer a variety of delicious and satisfying options to enjoy while following the Galveston Diet. Whether you prefer indulgent yet healthy treats, fruit-filled delights, or guilt-free chocolate confections, there's something for everyone to enjoy that will satisfy your sweet cravings and support your health and well-being. Experiment with different ingredients, flavors, and textures to create your own customized desserts that bring joy to your taste buds and nourish your body.

CHAPTER EIGHT

Meal Planning and Prep

Meal planning and preparation are essential components of a successful and sustainable approach to eating well. By taking the time to plan your meals and prepare ahead of time, you can save time, reduce stress, and make healthier choices throughout the week. Here are three key aspects of meal planning and prep to help you stay on track with your dietary goals:

Effective Meal Planning Strategies

Effective meal planning begins with setting realistic goals and creating a plan that fits your lifestyle and preferences. Here are some strategies to help you plan your meals effectively:

- **Set Realistic Goals**: Consider your dietary preferences, nutritional needs, and lifestyle factors when setting your meal planning goals. Aim for balanced meals that include a variety of foods from all food groups, and be realistic about your time, budget, and cooking skills.

- **Create a Weekly Menu**: Start by creating a weekly menu that includes breakfast, lunch, dinner, and snacks for each day of the week. Use a meal planning template or app to organize your meals and make it easier to stick to your plan.

- **Shop with a List**: Once you've planned your meals for the week, make a shopping list of all the ingredients you'll need.

Stick to your list to avoid impulse purchases and ensure you have everything on hand to prepare your meals.

- **Use Leftovers Wisely**: Incorporate leftovers into your meal plan to reduce waste and save time. Plan to cook larger batches of meals that can be enjoyed for multiple meals throughout the week, or repurpose leftovers into new dishes.

- **Be Flexible**: While it's important to have a plan, it's also important to be flexible and adaptable. Life can be unpredictable, so be prepared to make adjustments to your meal plan as needed based on changes in schedule, availability of ingredients, or dietary preferences.

Batch Cooking for Busy Weekdays

Batch cooking is a time-saving strategy that involves preparing large quantities of food ahead of time to enjoy throughout the week. Here are some tips for batch cooking:

- **Choose Batch-Friendly Recipes**: Look for recipes that are well-suited to batch cooking, such as soups, stews, casseroles, and grain salads. These dishes often improve in flavor over time and can be easily reheated for quick and convenient meals.

- **Invest in Storage Containers**: Invest in a variety of storage containers in different sizes to store your batch-cooked meals safely in the refrigerator or freezer. Choose containers that are microwave-safe and stackable for easy storage and reheating.

- **Prep Ingredients in Advance**: Spend some time on the weekend prepping ingredients such as chopping vegetables, marinating proteins, and cooking grains or legumes. Having these ingredients ready to go will make it easier to assemble meals quickly during the week.

- **Label and Date Your Meals**: To avoid confusion and ensure freshness, label and date your batch-cooked meals before storing them in the refrigerator or freezer. Use masking tape and a permanent marker to write the name of the dish and the date it was prepared.

- **Rotate Your Stock**: To prevent food waste, rotate your batch-cooked meals by using the oldest ones first and replenishing your stock with fresh batches as needed. Keep track of what you have on hand and plan your meals accordingly to avoid overstocking or running out of food.

Tips for Successful Meal Prepping

Meal prepping involves preparing ingredients or entire meals in advance to streamline the cooking process and make it easier to eat healthily throughout the week. Here are some tips for successful meal prepping:

- **Choose Versatile Ingredients**: Select ingredients that can be used in multiple dishes to maximize variety and minimize waste. For example, roast a batch of vegetables that can be used as a side dish, salad topping, or pizza topping throughout the week.

- **Plan Your Prep Sessions**: Set aside dedicated time each week for meal prepping, such as Sunday afternoon or Wednesday evening. Use this time to chop vegetables, cook grains, portion out snacks, and assemble meals for the week ahead.

- **Use Time-Saving Tools**: Invest in time-saving tools and appliances such as a slow cooker, Instant Pot, or food processor to streamline the meal prep process. These tools can help you cook large batches of food quickly and efficiently.

- **Organize Your Workspace**: Keep your kitchen organized and clutter-free to make meal prepping more efficient. Set up a designated workspace with all the necessary tools and ingredients within easy reach, and clean as you go to minimize mess and stress.

- **Divide and Conquer**: Break down meal prepping into smaller tasks to make it more manageable. For example, dedicate one day to prepping proteins, another day to chopping vegetables, and another day to assembling meals. This will help prevent burnout and keep you motivated to stick to your meal prep routine.

By incorporating effective meal planning and preparation strategies into your routine, you can save time, reduce stress, and make healthier choices throughout the week. Whether you're batch cooking for busy weekdays or prepping ingredients for quick and easy meals, these tips will help you stay on track with your dietary goals and enjoy delicious and nutritious meals every day.

CHAPTER NINE

Dining Out and Social Situations

Navigating restaurants and social gatherings while following the Galveston Diet can present unique challenges, but with the right strategies and mindset, you can still enjoy delicious meals and social interactions without compromising your health goals. Here are three key aspects to consider when dining out and navigating social situations:

Navigating Restaurants on the Galveston Diet

Eating out at restaurants can be enjoyable, but it can also present challenges when trying to stick to a specific dietary plan like the Galveston Diet. Here are some strategies to help you make healthier choices when dining out:

- **Plan Ahead**: Before heading to a restaurant, take some time to review the menu online, if available. Look for dishes that align with the principles of the Galveston Diet, such as protein-rich options, plenty of vegetables, and minimal processed ingredients.

- **Customize Your Order**: Don't be afraid to ask for modifications to suit your dietary preferences. For example, request grilled or baked options instead of fried, ask for sauces and dressings on the side, and substitute steamed vegetables or salad for starchy sides like fries or mashed potatoes.

- **Be Mindful of Portion Sizes**: Restaurant portions are often larger than what you might typically eat at home. Consider sharing a meal with a dining companion or asking for a half portion if available, or plan to take leftovers home for another meal.

- **Practice Moderation**: While it's okay to indulge occasionally, try to balance your meal by including plenty of vegetables and lean protein and limiting high-calorie or high-fat items. Enjoy your meal mindfully, savoring each bite and stopping when you feel satisfied.

- **Stay Hydrated**: Opt for water or herbal tea instead of sugary drinks or alcoholic beverages, which can add extra calories and contribute to overeating. Drinking plenty of water can also help you feel fuller and more satisfied throughout your meal.

Healthy Choices for Social Gatherings

Social gatherings often revolve around food, making it challenging to stick to your dietary goals. However, with a little planning and mindfulness, you can make healthier choices while still enjoying the company of friends and family. Here are some tips for making healthy choices at social gatherings:

- **Bring a Dish**: If you're attending a potluck or gathering where food will be served, consider bringing a dish that aligns with the Galveston Diet. This way, you'll have at least one option that you know you can enjoy guilt-free.

- **Focus on Protein and Vegetables**: When filling your plate, prioritize protein-rich options such as grilled chicken, fish, or tofu, along with plenty of vegetables. Fill up on these nutrient-dense foods first to help curb your appetite and prevent overindulging in less healthy options.

- **Practice Portion Control**: Be mindful of portion sizes and avoid mindlessly grazing on snacks or appetizers. Use a smaller plate if available, and aim to fill half of your plate with vegetables, a quarter with protein, and the remaining quarter with whole grains or other carbohydrates.

- **Limit Alcohol Intake**: Alcoholic beverages can be high in calories and can lower inhibitions, making it easier to overeat. If you choose to drink alcohol, do so in moderation and opt for lower-calorie options such as light beer, wine spritzers, or mixed drinks made with soda water or seltzer.

- **Stay Active**: Incorporate physical activity into your social gatherings by suggesting active outings such as hiking, biking, or playing sports. Not only will this help burn off extra calories, but it can also provide a fun and enjoyable way to spend time with friends and family.

Mindful Eating Techniques

Practicing mindful eating can help you become more aware of your eating habits and make healthier choices in any situation. Here are some techniques to help you eat more mindfully:

- **Slow Down**: Take your time to chew your food slowly and savor each bite. Put your fork down between bites, and take breaks to check in with your hunger and fullness cues.

- **Pay Attention to Hunger and Fullness**: Tune in to your body's hunger and fullness signals, and eat only when you're hungry and stop when you're satisfied. Avoid eating out of boredom, stress, or habit, and listen to your body's cues to guide your eating decisions.

- **Engage Your Senses**: Pay attention to the colors, textures, flavors, and aromas of your food as you eat. Notice the sensations of hunger and fullness, and how your body responds to different foods.

- **Practice Gratitude**: Take a moment before eating to express gratitude for the food on your plate and the nourishment it provides. Cultivating a sense of gratitude can help you appreciate your meals more fully and savor the experience of eating.

- **Be Non-Judgmental**: Approach your meals with curiosity and openness, without judgment or criticism. Be kind to yourself and acknowledge that it's okay to enjoy a variety of foods in moderation, without guilt or shame.

By incorporating these mindful eating techniques into your daily life, you can cultivate a healthier relationship with food and make more conscious choices that support your overall well-being. Whether dining out at restaurants or navigating social gatherings, mindfulness can help you stay on track with your dietary goals while still enjoying delicious meals and meaningful connections with others.

CHAPTER TEN

Maintaining Long-Term Success

Achieving long-term success on the Galveston Diet requires commitment, perseverance, and a positive mindset. While there may be challenges and setbacks along the way, staying motivated, overcoming obstacles, and celebrating achievements are essential for sustaining progress and reaching your health and wellness goals. Here are three key aspects to consider when maintaining long-term success:

Staying Motivated on Your Galveston Journey

Staying motivated is crucial for maintaining long-term success on the Galveston Diet. Here are some strategies to help you stay motivated throughout your journey:

- **Set Realistic Goals**: Set achievable goals that are specific, measurable, and attainable. Break larger goals into smaller, manageable steps, and track your progress over time to stay motivated and focused on your objectives.

- **Find Your Why**: Identify your reasons for wanting to follow the Galveston Diet and improve your health and well-being. Whether it's to feel more energized, lose weight, or reduce inflammation, connecting with your underlying motivations can help keep you inspired and committed to your goals.

- **Create a Support System**: Surround yourself with supportive friends, family members, or fellow Galveston Diet followers who can offer encouragement, accountability, and guidance along the way. Share your successes and challenges with others, and celebrate each other's progress together.

- **Visualize Success**: Visualize yourself achieving your goals and experiencing the positive outcomes of following the Galveston Diet. Use visualization techniques to imagine how you'll look, feel, and function at your best, and use these mental images as inspiration to keep you motivated and on track.

- **Reward Yourself**: Celebrate your achievements and milestones with non-food rewards that align with your health and wellness goals. Treat yourself to a new workout outfit, a relaxing massage, or a fun activity that brings you joy and reinforces your commitment to self-care.

Overcoming Challenges and Plateaus

Challenges and plateaus are inevitable on any health and wellness journey, but with resilience and determination, you can overcome obstacles and continue making progress. Here are some strategies to help you overcome challenges and plateaus on the Galveston Diet:

- **Stay Flexible**: Be prepared to adapt and adjust your approach as needed to overcome obstacles and navigate setbacks. If you encounter challenges or plateaus, reassess your goals, strategies, and habits, and make any necessary changes to keep moving forward.

- **Focus on Non-Scale Victories**: Instead of solely focusing on the number on the scale, celebrate non-scale victories such as improvements in energy levels, mood, sleep quality, and overall well-being. Recognize and appreciate the positive changes you're experiencing beyond just weight loss.

- **Reassess Your Habits**: Take a closer look at your dietary and lifestyle habits to identify any areas where you may be falling short or experiencing barriers to success. Make small, sustainable changes to your habits and routines to overcome obstacles and break through plateaus.

- **Seek Support and Guidance**: Don't hesitate to reach out for support and guidance from healthcare professionals, registered dietitians, or Galveston Diet coaches if you're struggling to overcome challenges or break through plateaus. They can provide personalized advice, encouragement, and resources to help you stay on track and achieve your goals.

- **Stay Patient and Persistent**: Remember that progress takes time, and setbacks are a natural part of the journey. Stay patient and persistent, and trust in your ability to overcome challenges and reach your long-term goals with perseverance and dedication.

Celebrating Achievements and Milestones

Celebrating achievements and milestones along the way is essential for maintaining motivation and reinforcing positive habits. Here are some ideas for celebrating your successes on the Galveston Diet:

- **Track Your Progress**: Keep track of your achievements and milestones, whether it's reaching a certain weight loss goal, fitting into a smaller clothing size, or improving your fitness level. Use a journal, calendar, or tracking app to monitor your progress and celebrate your accomplishments along the way.

- **Reward Yourself**: Treat yourself to a special reward or celebration when you achieve a significant milestone or goal. Whether it's a spa day, a weekend getaway, or a special meal at your favorite restaurant, choose rewards that align with your health and wellness goals and make you feel good about your achievements.

- **Share Your Successes**: Share your successes with others who support and encourage you, whether it's friends, family members, or fellow Galveston Diet followers. Celebrate your achievements together and use your accomplishments as inspiration to motivate others on their own health and wellness journeys.

- **Reflect on Your Journey**: Take time to reflect on how far you've come and acknowledge the hard work and dedication it took to reach your goals. Celebrate your progress and accomplishments, and use them as motivation to continue moving forward on your Galveston journey.

- **Set New Goals**: Once you've achieved a milestone or goal, set new challenges and objectives to keep yourself motivated and engaged. Whether it's running a 5K race, mastering a new healthy recipe, or reaching a new fitness milestone, setting new goals can help you stay focused and committed to your long-term success.

By staying motivated, overcoming challenges, and celebrating achievements, you can maintain long-term success on the Galveston Diet and continue to enjoy improved health, vitality, and well-being for years to come. Remember to stay patient, persistent, and positive, and celebrate every step of your journey toward optimal health and wellness.

CHAPTER 11

31 DAY MEAL PLAN

Day 1:

- Breakfast: Veggie omelet with spinach, mushrooms, and bell peppers cooked in olive oil.

- Lunch: Grilled chicken salad with mixed greens, cherry tomatoes, cucumbers, and a lemon vinaigrette.

- Dinner: Baked salmon with roasted asparagus and quinoa.

Day 2:

- Breakfast: Greek yogurt topped with blueberries and almonds.

- Lunch: Turkey and avocado wrap with lettuce, tomato, and whole grain tortilla.

- Dinner: Beef stir-fry with broccoli, bell peppers, and snap peas served over cauliflower rice.

Day 3:

- Breakfast: Smoothie made with kale, pineapple, banana, and almond milk.

- Lunch: Lentil soup with a side of mixed green salad.

- Dinner: Grilled shrimp skewers with zucchini noodles tossed in pesto.

Day 4:

- Breakfast: Scrambled eggs with diced tomatoes, onions, and feta cheese.

- Lunch: Tuna salad stuffed in a whole wheat pita pocket with spinach and cucumber slices.

- Dinner: Baked chicken thighs with roasted Brussels sprouts and sweet potatoes.

Day 5:

- Breakfast: Overnight oats made with rolled oats, almond milk, chia seeds, and topped with strawberries.

- Lunch: Quinoa salad with black beans, corn, diced peppers, and a lime-cilantro dressing.

- Dinner: Baked cod with steamed broccoli and wild rice.

Day 6:

- Breakfast: Whole grain toast topped with mashed avocado and sliced hard-boiled eggs.

- Lunch: Grilled vegetable wrap with hummus in a whole wheat tortilla.

- Dinner: Turkey meatballs served with marinara sauce over spaghetti squash.

Day 7:

- Breakfast: Cottage cheese mixed with sliced peaches and a sprinkle of cinnamon.

- Lunch: Chicken Caesar salad with romaine lettuce, grilled chicken breast, Parmesan cheese, and homemade dressing.

- Dinner: Baked tofu with stir-fried bok choy and brown rice.

Day 8:

- Breakfast: Spinach and feta crustless quiche.

- Lunch: Mixed bean salad with cherry tomatoes, cucumbers, and a lemon-tahini dressing.

- Dinner: Grilled steak with roasted cauliflower and a side of sautéed kale.

Day 9:

- Breakfast: Chia seed pudding topped with sliced strawberries and almonds.

- Lunch: Turkey and vegetable soup with a side of whole grain crackers.

- Dinner: Baked halibut with roasted asparagus and quinoa pilaf.

Day 10:

- Breakfast: Whole grain waffles topped with Greek yogurt and mixed berries.

- Lunch: Veggie wrap with hummus, roasted red peppers, cucumber, and shredded carrots.

- Dinner: Spaghetti squash with marinara sauce and turkey meatballs.

Day 11:

- Breakfast: Smoothie bowl made with mixed berries, banana, spinach, and almond milk, topped with granola and coconut flakes.

- Lunch: Quinoa and black bean stuffed bell peppers served with a side salad.

- Dinner: Grilled shrimp with roasted Brussels sprouts and sweet potato wedges.

Day 12:

- Breakfast: Avocado toast on whole grain bread topped with sliced tomatoes and a poached egg.

- Lunch: Lentil and vegetable curry with brown rice.

- Dinner: Baked chicken breasts with steamed broccoli and cauliflower mash.

Day 13:

- Breakfast: Cottage cheese mixed with diced pineapple and a drizzle of honey.

- Lunch: Turkey and avocado lettuce wraps with sliced bell peppers and cucumber.

- Dinner: Grilled salmon with roasted asparagus and wild rice pilaf.

Day 14:

- Breakfast: Scrambled eggs with sautéed spinach, mushrooms, and onions.

- Lunch: Chickpea salad with cherry tomatoes, cucumbers, feta cheese, and balsamic vinaigrette.

- Dinner: Stir-fried tofu with mixed vegetables served over cauliflower rice.

Day 15:

- Breakfast: Smoothie made with spinach, banana, almond butter, and almond milk.

- Lunch: Turkey and vegetable soup with a side of mixed greens salad.

- Dinner: Baked cod with roasted Brussels sprouts and quinoa.

Day 16:

- Breakfast: Greek yogurt parfait with layers of granola and mixed berries.

- Lunch: Quinoa salad with roasted vegetables and a lemon-tahini dressing.

- Dinner: Grilled chicken skewers with bell peppers and onions served with brown rice.

Day 17:

- Breakfast: Veggie scramble with diced bell peppers, onions, and tomatoes.

- Lunch: Tuna salad with mixed greens, cucumbers, and cherry tomatoes.

- Dinner: Baked turkey breast with steamed green beans and mashed sweet potatoes.

Day 18:

- Breakfast: Overnight oats with almond milk, sliced banana, and a sprinkle of cinnamon.

- Lunch: Lentil soup with a side of whole grain bread.

- Dinner: Baked tofu with stir-fried broccoli and carrots over brown rice.

Day 19:

- Breakfast: Whole grain toast topped with mashed avocado and sliced hard-boiled eggs.

- Lunch: Chicken Caesar salad with romaine lettuce, grilled chicken, and Parmesan cheese.

- Dinner: Baked salmon with roasted asparagus and quinoa.

Day 20:

- Breakfast: Smoothie bowl with mixed berries, banana, spinach, and almond milk, topped with granola and coconut flakes.

- Lunch: Turkey and avocado wrap with lettuce, tomato, and whole wheat tortilla.

- Dinner: Stir-fried shrimp with mixed vegetables served over cauliflower rice.

Day 21:

- Breakfast: Cottage cheese mixed with diced pineapple and a drizzle of honey.

- Lunch: Chickpea salad with cherry tomatoes, cucumbers, feta cheese, and balsamic vinaigrette.

- Dinner: Grilled chicken breasts with roasted Brussels sprouts and sweet potato wedges.

Day 22:

- Breakfast: Spinach and feta crustless quiche.

- Lunch: Mixed bean salad with cherry tomatoes, cucumbers, and a lemon-tahini dressing.

- Dinner: Grilled steak with roasted cauliflower and a side of sautéed kale.

Day 23:

- Breakfast: Chia seed pudding topped with sliced strawberries and almonds.

- Lunch: Turkey and vegetable soup with a side of whole grain crackers.

- Dinner: Baked halibut with roasted asparagus and quinoa pilaf.

Day 24:

- Breakfast: Whole grain waffles topped with Greek yogurt and mixed berries.

- Lunch: Veggie wrap with hummus, roasted red peppers, cucumber, and shredded carrots.

- Dinner: Spaghetti squash with marinara sauce and turkey meatballs.

Day 25:

- Breakfast: Smoothie bowl made with mixed berries, banana, spinach, and almond milk, topped with granola and coconut flakes.

- Lunch: Quinoa and black bean stuffed bell peppers served with a side salad.

- Dinner: Grilled shrimp with roasted Brussels sprouts and sweet potato wedges.

Day 26:

- Breakfast: Avocado toast on whole grain bread topped with sliced tomatoes and a poached egg.

- Lunch: Lentil and vegetable curry with brown rice.

- Dinner: Baked chicken breasts with steamed broccoli and cauliflower mash.

Day 27:

- Breakfast: Cottage cheese mixed with diced pineapple and a drizzle of honey.

- Lunch: Turkey and avocado lettuce wraps with sliced bell peppers and cucumber.

- Dinner: Grilled salmon with roasted asparagus and wild rice pilaf.

Day 28:

- Breakfast: Scrambled eggs with sautéed spinach, mushrooms, and onions.

- Lunch: Chickpea salad with cherry tomatoes, cucumbers, feta cheese, and balsamic vinaigrette.

- Dinner: Stir-fried tofu with mixed vegetables served over cauliflower rice.

Day 29:

- Breakfast: Greek yogurt parfait with layers of granola and mixed berries.

- Lunch: Turkey and vegetable soup with a side of mixed greens salad.

- Dinner: Baked cod with roasted Brussels sprouts and quinoa.

Day 30:

- Breakfast: Smoothie made with spinach, banana, almond butter, and almond milk.

- Lunch: Quinoa salad with roasted vegetables and a lemon-tahini dressing.

- Dinner: Grilled chicken skewers with bell peppers and onions served with brown rice.

Day 31:

- Breakfast: Veggie scramble with diced bell peppers, onions, and tomatoes.

- Lunch: Tuna salad with mixed greens, cucumbers, and cherry tomatoes.

- Dinner: Baked turkey breast with steamed green beans and mashed sweet potatoes.

BONUS

SOME ESSENTIAL DIETS FOR HEALTHY LIVING

Turkey Diet

Definition: The turkey diet involves incorporating turkey as a lean and protein-rich source into meals. Turkey is low in fat and calories while being high in protein, making it an excellent choice for those looking to increase their protein intake while managing their calorie intake. It also provides essential nutrients such as vitamins B6 and B12, niacin, zinc, and selenium.

Ingredients:

- **Turkey:** The star ingredient, rich in protein and low in fat, serves as the foundation of this diet.

- **Vegetables:** Pair turkey with a variety of vegetables such as spinach, kale, broccoli, or bell peppers for added nutrients, fiber, and flavor.

- **Whole Grains:** Serve turkey alongside whole grains like quinoa, brown rice, or whole wheat pasta for sustained energy and additional fiber.

- **Healthy Fats:** Incorporate sources of healthy fats such as olive oil, avocado, nuts, or seeds to enhance satiety and nutrient absorption.

- **Herbs and Spices:** Flavor turkey dishes with herbs, spices, and seasonings like garlic, rosemary, thyme, or paprika to enhance taste and aroma.

Instructions:

1. **Grilled Turkey Breast:** Grill turkey breast seasoned with herbs and spices until cooked through for a simple and delicious main dish that's perfect for summer barbecues.

2. **Turkey Stir-Fry:** Stir-fry sliced turkey breast with vegetables, garlic, ginger, and soy sauce for a quick and flavorful Asian-inspired dish that's perfect for busy weeknights.

3. **Turkey Salad:** Toss sliced turkey breast with mixed greens, avocado, walnuts, and a balsamic vinaigrette for a refreshing and nutrient-rich salad that's perfect for lunch or dinner.

4. **Turkey Wrap:** Wrap sliced turkey breast with lettuce, tomato, avocado, and hummus in a whole grain tortilla for a satisfying and portable meal option that's perfect for lunch or snacks.

5. **Turkey Chili:** Simmer ground turkey with tomatoes, beans, onions, and spices until flavors meld together for a hearty and nutritious chili that's perfect for cold weather or game days.

Walnuts Diet

Definition: The walnuts diet involves incorporating walnuts as a nutritious and heart-healthy nut into meals or snacks. Walnuts are rich in omega-3 fatty acids, antioxidants, vitamins (such as vitamin E), minerals (such as magnesium and copper), and fiber, making them a valuable addition to any diet.

Ingredients:

- **Walnuts:** The star ingredient, rich in omega-3 fatty acids, antioxidants, vitamins, minerals, and fiber, serves as the foundation of this diet.

- **Other Nuts and Seeds:** Pair walnuts with other nuts or seeds such as almonds, pecans, or chia seeds for added texture, flavor, and nutritional benefits.

- **Fruits:** Enjoy walnuts with fruits like apples, berries, or pears for a sweet and savory snack option that's rich in flavor and nutrients.

- **Whole Grains:** Serve walnuts alongside whole grains like oats, quinoa, or whole grain bread for added fiber and sustained energy.

- **Dairy or Dairy Alternatives:** Combine walnuts with Greek yogurt, almond milk, or cottage cheese for a creamy and nutritious breakfast or snack option.

Instructions:

1. **Raw Walnuts:** Enjoy raw walnuts on their own as a quick and convenient snack option that's packed with omega-3 fatty acids, antioxidants, and fiber.

2. **Walnut Trail Mix:** Combine walnuts with other nuts, seeds, dried fruits, and a sprinkle of dark chocolate chips for a flavorful and energizing trail mix that's perfect for hiking or snacking on the go.

3. **Walnut Salad:** Sprinkle chopped walnuts over mixed greens, sliced strawberries, goat cheese, and a balsamic vinaigrette for a refreshing and nutrient-rich salad that's perfect for lunch or dinner.

4. **Walnut Oatmeal:** Stir chopped walnuts into cooked oatmeal along with cinnamon, maple syrup, and a splash of almond milk for a hearty and satisfying breakfast option that's perfect for chilly mornings.

5. **Walnut Pesto:** Blend walnuts with basil, garlic, olive oil, Parmesan cheese, and lemon juice until smooth for a delicious and flavorful pesto sauce that's perfect for tossing with pasta, spreading on sandwiches, or topping grilled meats.

Watermelon Diet

Definition: The watermelon diet involves incorporating watermelon as a refreshing and hydrating fruit into meals or snacks. Watermelon is low in calories, high in water content, and packed with vitamins (such as vitamin C and vitamin A), minerals (such as potassium), and antioxidants (such as lycopene), making it a delicious and nutritious addition to any diet.

Ingredients:

- **Watermelon:** The star ingredient, rich in water, vitamins, minerals, and antioxidants, serves as the foundation of this diet.

- **Other Fruits:** Pair watermelon with other fruits such as berries, oranges, or kiwi for added flavor, sweetness, and variety.

- **Leafy Greens:** Toss watermelon chunks with mixed greens, feta cheese, mint, and a balsamic vinaigrette for a refreshing and nutrient-rich salad.

- **Mint:** Add fresh mint leaves to watermelon salads, smoothies, or agua frescas for a burst of freshness and flavor.

- **Citrus:** Squeeze lime or lemon juice over watermelon slices for a tangy and refreshing twist.

Instructions:

1. **Fresh Watermelon:** Enjoy chilled watermelon slices on their own as a refreshing and hydrating snack.

2. **Watermelon Smoothie:** Blend watermelon chunks with lime juice, mint leaves, and a splash of coconut water for a refreshing and hydrating smoothie that's perfect for hot days.

3. **Watermelon Salad:** Combine watermelon cubes with feta cheese, cucumber slices, red onion, and fresh mint leaves tossed in a lime vinaigrette for a refreshing and flavorful salad that's perfect for summer.

4. **Watermelon Gazpacho:** Blend watermelon chunks with tomatoes, cucumber, red bell pepper, red onion, garlic, and jalapeno until smooth, then chill for a refreshing and hydrating soup option that's perfect for warm weather.

5. **Watermelon Salsa:** Dice watermelon and combine with diced tomatoes, red onion, jalapeno, cilantro, lime juice, and a pinch of salt for a sweet and spicy salsa that's perfect for serving with grilled fish or chicken.

Zucchini Diet

Definition: The zucchini diet involves incorporating zucchini as a nutritious and versatile vegetable into meals. Zucchini is low in calories, rich in fiber, vitamins (such as vitamin C and vitamin K), minerals (such as potassium and manganese), and antioxidants, making it a valuable addition to any diet.

Ingredients:

- **Zucchini:** The star ingredient, rich in fiber, vitamins, minerals, and antioxidants, serves as the foundation of this diet.

- **Other Vegetables:** Pair zucchini with a variety of vegetables such as tomatoes, bell peppers, onions, or mushrooms for added flavor, texture, and nutrients.

- **Whole Grains:** Serve zucchini alongside whole grains like quinoa, brown rice, or whole wheat pasta for added fiber and sustained energy.

- **Proteins:** Pair zucchini with proteins like grilled chicken, tofu, chickpeas, or shrimp to create balanced and satisfying meals.

- **Herbs and Spices:** Flavor zucchini dishes with herbs, spices, and seasonings like garlic, basil, oregano, or red pepper flakes to enhance taste and aroma.

Instructions:

1. **Grilled Zucchini:** Slice zucchini lengthwise, brush with olive oil, sprinkle with salt and pepper, then grill until tender and slightly charred for a simple and delicious side dish that's perfect for summer barbecues.

2. **Zucchini Noodles:** Spiralize zucchini into noodles and toss with marinara sauce, garlic, and basil for a light and flavorful pasta alternative that's perfect for low-carb or gluten-free diets.

3. **Stuffed Zucchini:** Hollow out zucchini halves and fill with a mixture of cooked quinoa, vegetables, herbs, and cheese, then bake until tender for a delicious and nutritious vegetarian entree option.

4. **Zucchini Stir-Fry:** Stir-fry sliced zucchini with other vegetables, tofu, or shrimp in a savory sauce made with soy sauce, garlic, ginger, and sesame oil for a quick and flavorful Asian-inspired dish that's perfect for weeknight dinners.

5. **Zucchini Fritters:** Grate zucchini and mix with eggs, breadcrumbs, Parmesan cheese, and herbs, then pan-fry until golden and crispy for a delicious and nutritious appetizer or snack option.

Almonds Diet

Definition: The almonds diet is a dietary approach that incorporates almonds as a primary component of meals or snacks. It often involves consuming almonds in various forms throughout the day to promote health and potentially aid in weight management.

Ingredients: Almonds are the central ingredient in the almonds diet. They are rich in healthy fats, protein, fiber, vitamins, and minerals. Additionally, the diet may include other foods such as fruits, vegetables, lean proteins, and whole grains to ensure a balanced nutrient intake.

Instructions:

1. **Incorporate Almonds Into Meals:** Include almonds in your breakfast, lunch, dinner, and snacks. For breakfast, add almonds to your cereal, yogurt, or oatmeal. For lunch and dinner, sprinkle almonds over salads or incorporate them into stir-fries and grain dishes.

2. **Snack on Almonds:** Keep a handful of almonds as a convenient and nutritious snack option. You can enjoy them on their own or pair them with fruits like apples or berries.

3. **Portion Control:** While almonds are nutritious, they are also calorie-dense. Practice portion control to avoid overconsumption, especially if your goal is weight management.

4. **Variety:** Experiment with different almond varieties such as raw, roasted, or flavored almonds to keep your meals interesting and flavorful.

5. **Stay Hydrated:** Drink plenty of water throughout the day, as almonds are naturally low in water content and hydration is essential for overall health and digestion.

Avocado Diet

Definition: The avocado diet emphasizes the inclusion of avocados as a significant component of meals. Avocados are known for their rich nutrient profile, including healthy fats, fiber, vitamins, and minerals.

Ingredients: Avocados are the main ingredient in the avocado diet. They can be used in various forms, including sliced, mashed, or blended into recipes. Other ingredients may include vegetables, lean proteins, whole grains, and healthy fats.

Instructions:

1. **Incorporate Avocados Into Meals:** Include avocados in your meals throughout the day. Add sliced avocado to sandwiches, wraps, and salads. Use mashed avocado as a spread on toast or as a topping for grilled proteins.

2. **Avocado Smoothies:** Blend avocado with fruits like bananas, berries, or spinach to create creamy and nutritious smoothies. You can also add protein powder or nut milk for an extra nutritional boost.

3. **Healthy Fats:** Avocados are rich in monounsaturated fats, which are beneficial for heart health. However, be mindful of portion sizes, as avocados are calorie-dense.

4. **Balanced Diet:** While avocados are nutritious, it's essential to maintain a balanced diet by including a variety of foods from all food groups.

5. **Enjoy in Moderation:** Avocados can be a healthy addition to your diet, but moderation is key. Monitor your portion sizes

to avoid excessive calorie intake, especially if you're watching your weight.

Black Beans Diet

Definition: The black beans diet revolves around integrating black beans as a staple in meals to boost nutrition and promote overall health. Black beans are a type of legume rich in protein, fiber, vitamins, and minerals, making them a valuable addition to various dietary plans.

Ingredients:

- **Black Beans:** The primary ingredient, rich in protein and fiber, forms the cornerstone of this diet.

- **Vegetables:** Complement meals with a variety of vegetables for added nutrients and flavor.

- **Grains:** Incorporate whole grains like brown rice, quinoa, or whole wheat pasta for a balanced meal.

- **Lean Proteins:** Include lean proteins such as chicken, fish, or tofu to enhance the protein content and diversity of nutrients in your diet.

- **Herbs and Spices:** Flavor dishes with herbs, spices, and seasonings to enhance taste without relying on excessive salt or unhealthy additives.

Instructions:

1. **Include Black Beans in Meals:** Incorporate black beans into various meals, such as salads, soups, stews, burritos, tacos, or grain bowls.

2. **Diversify Your Recipes:** Experiment with different recipes and cuisines that feature black beans as a central ingredient. Explore Mexican, Cuban, or Southwestern-inspired dishes for variety.

3. **Combine with Complementary Foods:** Pair black beans with complementary foods to create balanced and satisfying meals. For example, combine black beans with rice for a complete protein source or add them to salads for extra fiber and protein.

4. **Watch Portion Sizes:** While black beans are nutritious, they are also calorie-dense. Be mindful of portion sizes, especially if you're watching your calorie intake or managing your weight.

5. **Prepare in Advance:** Cook a batch of black beans in advance and store them in the fridge or freezer for quick and convenient meal prep throughout the week.

Blueberries Diet

Definition: The blueberries diet emphasizes the consumption of blueberries as a primary source of antioxidants, vitamins, and fiber. Blueberries are renowned for their potential health benefits, including improved cognitive function, heart health, and management of blood sugar levels.

Ingredients:

- **Blueberries:** The star ingredient, packed with antioxidants and nutrients.

- **Other Fruits:** Incorporate a variety of fruits alongside blueberries to diversify nutrient intake and add natural sweetness to meals and snacks.

- **Dairy or Non-Dairy Products:** Pair blueberries with yogurt, milk, or dairy alternatives like almond milk for a nutritious breakfast or snack option.

- **Whole Grains:** Include whole grains such as oats, barley, or whole wheat toast to create balanced meals that provide sustained energy.

- **Nuts and Seeds:** Add nuts or seeds like almonds, walnuts, or chia seeds for additional nutrients and texture.

Instructions:

1. **Enjoy Blueberries Daily:** Aim to include blueberries in your daily diet by adding them to breakfasts, snacks, or desserts.

2. **Incorporate into Meals:** Add blueberries to oatmeal, yogurt bowls, smoothies, salads, or baked goods like muffins and pancakes.

3. **Mix with Other Fruits:** Combine blueberries with other fruits in salads, fruit bowls, or as toppings for yogurt or cereal to increase variety and nutrient intake.

4. **Experiment with Recipes:** Explore different recipes that feature blueberries as a central ingredient, such as blueberry chia pudding, blueberry smoothie bowls, or blueberry quinoa salad.

5. **Frozen Blueberries:** Keep frozen blueberries on hand to enjoy year-round and add them to recipes or snacks whenever fresh blueberries are not available.

Broccoli Diet

Definition: The broccoli diet focuses on incorporating broccoli as a prominent component of meals due to its high nutritional value. Broccoli is packed with vitamins, minerals, fiber, and antioxidants, making it a popular choice for those seeking to improve their overall health and well-being.

Ingredients:

- **Broccoli:** The main ingredient, rich in vitamin C, vitamin K, folate, and fiber.

- **Lean Proteins:** Include lean proteins such as chicken, fish, tofu, or legumes to create balanced meals.

- **Whole Grains:** Pair broccoli with whole grains like quinoa, brown rice, or whole wheat pasta for added fiber and nutrients.

- **Healthy Fats:** Incorporate sources of healthy fats like avocado, olive oil, nuts, or seeds to enhance nutrient absorption and satiety.

- **Herbs and Spices:** Flavor dishes with herbs, spices, and seasonings to enhance taste without relying on excessive salt or unhealthy additives.

Instructions:

1. **Include Broccoli in Meals:** Incorporate broccoli into various meals, such as stir-fries, salads, soups, casseroles, or as a side dish.

2. **Steam, Roast, or Saute:** Experiment with different cooking methods to prepare broccoli, such as steaming, roasting, or sautéing, to enhance flavor and texture.

3. **Pair with Protein:** Combine broccoli with lean proteins to create balanced and satisfying meals that provide a complete source of nutrients.

4. **Add Variety:** Explore different recipes and flavor combinations to keep meals interesting and enjoyable. Consider adding broccoli to pasta dishes, grain bowls, or frittatas.

5. **Meal Prep:** Prepare broccoli in advance and store it in the fridge for quick and convenient meal prep throughout the week. You can also freeze broccoli for longer-term storage.

Brussels Sprouts Diet

Definition: The Brussels sprouts diet centers around incorporating Brussels sprouts as a key ingredient in meals to boost nutrition and add variety to the diet. Brussels sprouts are a nutrient-dense vegetable rich in vitamins, minerals, fiber, and antioxidants, making them a valuable addition to any healthy eating plan.

Ingredients:

- **Brussels Sprouts:** The star ingredient, packed with vitamin K, vitamin C, folate, and fiber.

- **Other Vegetables:** Combine Brussels sprouts with other vegetables such as carrots, bell peppers, or cauliflower for added nutrients and flavor.

- **Proteins:** Pair Brussels sprouts with proteins like chicken, turkey, salmon, or tofu to create balanced and satisfying meals.

- **Whole Grains:** Serve Brussels sprouts alongside whole grains like quinoa, barley, or brown rice for added fiber and nutrients.

- **Healthy Fats:** Incorporate sources of healthy fats like olive oil, avocado, nuts, or seeds to enhance nutrient absorption and satiety.

Instructions:

1. **Prepare Brussels Sprouts:** Trim Brussels sprouts and cut them in half before cooking to ensure even cooking and enhanced flavor.

2. **Roast or Saute:** Roast Brussels sprouts in the oven with olive oil, garlic, and your favorite herbs and spices for a crispy and flavorful side dish. Alternatively, sauté Brussels sprouts with onions, garlic, and balsamic vinegar for a savory and delicious option.

3. **Pair with Protein:** Combine Brussels sprouts with lean proteins to create balanced meals that provide a complete source of nutrients. Try adding roasted Brussels sprouts to salads, grain bowls, or pasta dishes with grilled chicken or tofu.

4. **Experiment with Flavors:** Explore different flavor combinations by adding ingredients like bacon, maple syrup, Parmesan cheese, or dried cranberries to Brussels sprouts for added depth and complexity.

5. **Meal Prep:** Prepare a large batch of roasted Brussels sprouts and store them in the fridge for easy meal prep throughout

the week. You can also freeze cooked Brussels sprouts for longer-term storage and convenience.

Chicken Diet

Definition: The chicken diet revolves around incorporating chicken as a primary source of lean protein in meals. Chicken is versatile, low in fat (especially if you remove the skin), and packed with essential nutrients like protein, vitamins, and minerals, making it a popular choice for those aiming to maintain or build muscle mass while keeping calorie intake in check.

Ingredients:

- **Chicken:** The main ingredient, providing a lean source of protein.

- **Vegetables:** Pair chicken with a variety of vegetables to increase fiber intake and add essential vitamins and minerals to meals.

- **Whole Grains:** Serve chicken alongside whole grains like brown rice, quinoa, or whole wheat pasta for sustained energy and additional fiber.

- **Healthy Fats:** Incorporate sources of healthy fats such as avocado, olive oil, nuts, or seeds to enhance satiety and nutrient absorption.

- **Herbs and Spices:** Flavor chicken dishes with herbs, spices, and seasonings to add depth and complexity to the flavors without relying on excessive salt or unhealthy additives.

Instructions:

1. **Choose Lean Cuts:** Opt for lean cuts of chicken such as chicken breast or skinless chicken thighs to minimize saturated fat intake.

2. **Grill, Bake, or Broil:** Cook chicken using healthy cooking methods like grilling, baking, or broiling to minimize added fats and calories.

3. **Add Flavor:** Marinate chicken with herbs, spices, citrus juice, or yogurt-based marinades to infuse flavor and tenderize the meat before cooking.

4. **Pair with Vegetables:** Serve chicken with a generous portion of vegetables to create balanced and nutritious meals. Try roasted vegetables, stir-fried veggies, or a colorful salad.

5. **Meal Prep:** Prepare batches of grilled or baked chicken in advance and portion them out for easy meal prep throughout the week. You can also freeze cooked chicken for longer-term storage and convenience.

Chia Seeds Diet

Definition: The chia seeds diet incorporates chia seeds as a nutritional powerhouse into meals to boost fiber, protein, omega-3 fatty acids, and various micronutrients. Chia seeds are versatile and can be easily added to a wide range of dishes, making them a convenient addition to any diet.

Ingredients:

- **Chia Seeds:** The star ingredient, rich in fiber, protein, omega-3 fatty acids, and antioxidants.

- **Liquid:** Mix chia seeds with liquids such as water, milk (dairy or plant-based), yogurt, or fruit juice to create chia seed pudding or beverages.

- **Fruits:** Pair chia seeds with fruits like berries, bananas, or mangoes for added flavor, sweetness, and additional nutrients.

- **Nuts and Seeds:** Combine chia seeds with nuts or seeds such as almonds, walnuts, or pumpkin seeds for added texture and nutritional variety.

- **Sweeteners (Optional):** Add natural sweeteners like honey, maple syrup, or agave nectar if desired, but keep in mind the added sugar content.

Instructions:

1. **Chia Seed Pudding:** Mix chia seeds with your choice of liquid (e.g., almond milk) and sweetener (if desired), then let it sit in the fridge overnight to thicken into a pudding-like consistency. Serve with fresh fruit or nuts for added flavor and texture.

2. **Smoothies:** Blend chia seeds into smoothies along with fruits, leafy greens, protein powder, and your choice of liquid for a nutritious and filling beverage.

3. **Salads and Yogurt:** Sprinkle chia seeds over salads or yogurt bowls to add crunch, fiber, and omega-3 fatty acids.

4. **Baking:** Incorporate chia seeds into baked goods like muffins, bread, or energy bars for added nutrition and texture. Chia seeds can be used as an egg substitute in vegan baking recipes.

5. **Hydration:** Mix chia seeds into water or flavored beverages to create a hydrating chia seed drink. The seeds absorb liquid and develop a gel-like consistency, providing sustained hydration and a boost of nutrients.

Cottage Cheese Diet

Definition: The cottage cheese diet involves incorporating cottage cheese as a central component of meals or snacks. Cottage cheese is a low-fat dairy product rich in protein, calcium, and other essential nutrients. It's often used by individuals aiming to increase protein intake, promote muscle growth, and support weight loss or management.

Ingredients:

- **Cottage Cheese:** The primary ingredient, rich in protein and calcium, serves as the foundation of this diet.

- **Fruits:** Pair cottage cheese with fruits like berries, peaches, or pineapple for added flavor, natural sweetness, and additional vitamins and minerals.

- **Vegetables:** Combine cottage cheese with vegetables such as cucumbers, tomatoes, or bell peppers for a savory twist and increased fiber content.

- **Whole Grains:** Serve cottage cheese alongside whole grains like whole wheat crackers or bread for added fiber and sustained energy.

- **Herbs and Spices:** Flavor cottage cheese with herbs, spices, or seasonings like black pepper, dill, or chives to enhance taste without relying on excessive salt or unhealthy additives.

Instructions:

1. **Simple Snack:** Enjoy cottage cheese on its own as a quick and convenient snack option.

2. **Fruit Parfait:** Layer cottage cheese with your favorite fruits and a drizzle of honey or maple syrup to create a delicious and nutritious parfait.

3. **Salad Topping:** Use cottage cheese as a topping for salads instead of traditional dressings. It adds creaminess and protein to your salad while keeping the calorie count lower.

4. **Smoothies:** Blend cottage cheese into smoothies along with fruits, leafy greens, and your choice of liquid for a protein-rich beverage.

5. **Stuffed Vegetables:** Use cottage cheese as a filling for stuffed vegetables like bell peppers or tomatoes, along with herbs, spices, and other veggies for added flavor and nutrition.

Cucumbers Diet

Definition: The cucumbers diet emphasizes the consumption of cucumbers as a primary vegetable in meals or snacks. Cucumbers are low in calories, refreshing, and hydrating, making them an excellent choice for those looking to increase vegetable intake, support hydration, and promote weight loss or management.

Ingredients:

- **Cucumbers:** The star ingredient, low in calories and high in water content, serves as the foundation of this diet.

- **Dressing or Dip:** Pair cucumbers with healthy dressings or dips such as hummus, Greek yogurt-based dips, or vinaigrettes for added flavor and creaminess.

- **Proteins:** Combine cucumbers with protein sources like grilled chicken, tofu, or chickpeas to create balanced and satisfying meals.

- **Whole Grains:** Serve cucumbers alongside whole grains like quinoa, brown rice, or farro for added fiber and sustained energy.

- **Herbs and Spices:** Flavor cucumbers with herbs, spices, or seasonings like mint, dill, or lemon zest to enhance taste and aroma.

Instructions:

1. **Simple Snack:** Enjoy sliced cucumbers on their own as a refreshing and hydrating snack option.

2. **Salads:** Incorporate cucumbers into salads alongside other vegetables, greens, proteins, and grains for a nutritious and filling meal.

3. **Cucumber Cups:** Use cucumber slices or hollowed-out cucumber halves as cups to hold fillings like tuna salad, chicken salad, or hummus for a fun and creative appetizer or snack.

4. **Pickles:** Make homemade pickles by soaking cucumber slices in a mixture of vinegar, water, salt, and spices for a tangy and crunchy snack.

5. **Cucumber Water:** Infuse water with cucumber slices and fresh herbs like mint or basil for a refreshing and hydrating beverage option.

Egg Diet

Definition: The egg diet involves incorporating eggs as a primary source of protein in meals. Eggs are nutrient-dense, rich in high-quality protein, vitamins, minerals, and healthy fats. This diet is often used for weight loss, muscle building, or as part of a balanced eating plan.

Ingredients:

- **Eggs:** The main ingredient, providing high-quality protein, essential vitamins (such as vitamin B12 and vitamin D), and minerals (such as iron and selenium).

- **Vegetables:** Pair eggs with a variety of vegetables like spinach, bell peppers, tomatoes, or mushrooms for added fiber, vitamins, and minerals.

- **Whole Grains:** Serve eggs alongside whole grains such as whole wheat toast, quinoa, or oatmeal for sustained energy and additional fiber.

- **Healthy Fats:** Incorporate sources of healthy fats like avocado, olive oil, nuts, or seeds to enhance satiety and nutrient absorption.

- **Herbs and Spices:** Flavor egg dishes with herbs, spices, and seasonings like black pepper, paprika, or fresh herbs to add depth and complexity to the flavors.

Instructions:

1. **Basic Preparation:** Enjoy eggs cooked in various ways, such as boiled, poached, scrambled, fried (using minimal oil), or baked, depending on personal preference.

2. **Omelets:** Make omelets by whisking eggs with vegetables, cheese, and herbs, then cooking them in a skillet until set. Customize omelets with your favorite fillings for a nutritious and satisfying meal.

3. **Frittatas:** Bake eggs with vegetables and cheese in a frittata for a simple and versatile dish that can be enjoyed for breakfast, lunch, or dinner.

4. **Egg Salad:** Prepare egg salad by mixing chopped hard-boiled eggs with Greek yogurt, mustard, celery, and spices. Serve on whole grain bread or lettuce wraps for a protein-rich meal.

5. **Meal Prep:** Boil a batch of eggs in advance and store them in the fridge for easy meal prep throughout the week. Hard-

boiled eggs make a convenient and portable snack or addition to salads and sandwiches.

Pear Diet

Definition: The pear diet involves incorporating pears as a primary source of vitamins, minerals, and fiber into meals or snacks. Pears are rich in vitamin C, vitamin K, potassium, and dietary fiber, making them a nutritious and delicious addition to any diet.

Ingredients:

- **Pears:** The star ingredient, rich in vitamins, minerals, and fiber, serves as the foundation of this diet.

- **Other Fruits:** Pair pears with other fruits such as apples, berries, or grapes for added flavor, sweetness, and variety.

- **Greek Yogurt:** Combine sliced pears with Greek yogurt for a creamy and nutritious breakfast or snack option that's rich in protein and probiotics.

- **Nuts and Seeds:** Sprinkle chopped pears over nuts or seeds like almonds, walnuts, or chia seeds for added texture, healthy fats, and nutritional variety.

- **Whole Grains:** Serve pears alongside whole grains like oatmeal, quinoa, or whole grain bread for added fiber and sustained energy.

Instructions:

1. **Fresh Pears:** Enjoy ripe pears on their own by slicing them and removing the core for a refreshing and nutritious snack.

2. **Pear Smoothie:** Blend pear slices with other fruits, Greek yogurt, nut milk, and a scoop of protein powder for a creamy and refreshing smoothie that's packed with vitamins, minerals, and protein.

3. **Pear Salad:** Combine sliced pears with mixed greens, goat cheese, toasted nuts, and a balsamic vinaigrette for a refreshing and nutrient-rich salad that's perfect for lunch or dinner.

4. **Pear Tart:** Bake sliced pears on top of puff pastry with a sprinkle of cinnamon and sugar for a simple and elegant dessert option that's perfect for entertaining.

5. **Pear Sauce:** Cook sliced pears with a splash of water, lemon juice, and cinnamon until soft, then puree until smooth for a delicious and versatile sauce that can be served with pancakes, yogurt, or oatmeal.

Pineapple Diet

Definition: The pineapple diet involves incorporating pineapple as a primary source of vitamins, minerals, and enzymes into meals or snacks. Pineapple is rich in vitamin C, manganese, bromelain (an enzyme with anti-inflammatory properties), and dietary fiber, making it a flavorful and nutritious addition to any diet.

Ingredients:

- **Pineapple:** The star ingredient, rich in vitamins, minerals, enzymes, and fiber, serves as the foundation of this diet.

- **Other Fruits:** Pair pineapple with other fruits such as mango, kiwi, or papaya for added flavor, sweetness, and variety.

- **Greek Yogurt:** Combine pineapple chunks with Greek yogurt for a creamy and nutritious breakfast or snack option that's rich in protein and probiotics.

- **Nuts and Seeds:** Sprinkle chopped pineapple over nuts or seeds like macadamia nuts, coconut flakes, or hemp seeds for added texture, healthy fats, and nutritional variety.

- **Leafy Greens:** Toss pineapple chunks with mixed greens, avocado, nuts, and a citrus vinaigrette for a refreshing and nutrient-rich salad.

Instructions:

1. **Fresh Pineapple:** Enjoy ripe pineapple chunks on their own as a refreshing and nutritious snack.

2. **Pineapple Smoothie:** Blend pineapple chunks with other fruits, Greek yogurt, nut milk, and a scoop of protein powder

for a creamy and tropical smoothie that's packed with vitamins, minerals, and protein.

3. **Pineapple Salsa:** Dice pineapple and combine with chopped tomatoes, onions, cilantro, jalapeno, lime juice, and a pinch of salt for a flavorful and vibrant salsa that pairs well with grilled fish or chicken.

4. **Grilled Pineapple:** Grill pineapple slices until caramelized and slightly charred for a sweet and smoky side dish or dessert option that's perfect for summer barbecues.

5. **Pineapple Stir-Fry:** Stir-fry pineapple chunks with vegetables, tofu, or shrimp in a sweet and tangy sauce for a quick and flavorful Asian-inspired dish that's perfect for weeknight dinners.

Pistachios Diet

Definition: The pistachios diet involves incorporating pistachios as a nutritious and versatile nut into meals or snacks. Pistachios are rich in protein, healthy fats, fiber, vitamins (such as vitamin B6 and vitamin E), minerals (such as potassium and magnesium), and antioxidants, making them a valuable addition to any diet.

Ingredients:

- **Pistachios:** The star ingredient, rich in protein, healthy fats, fiber, vitamins, minerals, and antioxidants, serves as the foundation of this diet.

- **Other Nuts and Seeds:** Pair pistachios with other nuts or seeds such as almonds, walnuts, or pumpkin seeds for added texture, variety, and nutritional benefits.

- **Fruits:** Enjoy pistachios with fruits like apples, berries, or oranges for a sweet and savory snack option that's rich in flavor and nutrients.

- **Whole Grains:** Serve pistachios alongside whole grains like quinoa, brown rice, or whole grain crackers for added fiber and sustained energy.

- **Spices and Seasonings:** Flavor pistachios with spices and seasonings like chili powder, garlic powder, or cinnamon for a savory or sweet twist, depending on your preference.

Instructions:

1. **Raw Pistachios:** Enjoy raw pistachios on their own as a quick and convenient snack option that's packed with protein, healthy fats, and fiber.

2. **Roasted Pistachios:** Roast pistachios in the oven with a sprinkle of salt, garlic powder, or other seasonings for a crunchy and savory snack option that's perfect for movie nights or gatherings.

3. **Pistachio Butter:** Make pistachio butter by blending pistachios with a touch of honey or maple syrup until

smooth for a creamy and nutritious spread that's perfect for toast, fruit, or oatmeal.

4. **Pistachio Trail Mix:** Combine pistachios with other nuts, seeds, dried fruits, and a sprinkle of dark chocolate chips for a flavorful and energizing trail mix that's perfect for hiking or snacking on the go.

5. **Pistachio-Crusted Chicken:** Coat chicken breasts with crushed pistachios and breadcrumbs, then bake until golden and crispy for a delicious and nutritious entree option that's perfect for dinner.

Quinoa Diet

Definition: The quinoa diet involves incorporating quinoa as a nutritious and versatile whole grain into meals to boost protein, fiber, and nutrient intake. Quinoa is a complete protein, meaning it contains all nine essential amino acids, making it an excellent plant-based protein source for vegetarians and vegans.

Ingredients:

- **Quinoa:** The star ingredient, rich in protein, fiber, vitamins (such as B vitamins), minerals (such as iron and magnesium), and antioxidants, serves as the foundation of this diet.

- **Vegetables:** Pair quinoa with a variety of vegetables such as bell peppers, tomatoes, spinach, or avocado for added flavor, texture, and nutrients.

- **Proteins:** Serve quinoa alongside proteins like grilled chicken, tofu, chickpeas, or shrimp to create balanced and satisfying meals.

- **Healthy Fats:** Incorporate sources of healthy fats such as olive oil, avocado, nuts, or seeds to enhance satiety and nutrient absorption.

- **Herbs and Spices:** Flavor quinoa dishes with herbs, spices, and seasonings like garlic, onion powder, cumin, or paprika to enhance taste and aroma.

Instructions:

1. **Quinoa Salad:** Toss cooked quinoa with diced vegetables, herbs, nuts, and a lemon vinaigrette for a refreshing and nutrient-rich salad that's perfect for lunch or dinner.

2. **Quinoa Bowl:** Build a quinoa bowl with cooked quinoa as the base, then top with proteins, vegetables, avocado, and a drizzle of tahini or salsa for a satisfying and customizable meal option.

3. **Quinoa Stir-Fry:** Stir-fry cooked quinoa with vegetables, tofu, or shrimp in a savory sauce made with soy sauce, garlic, ginger, and sesame oil for a quick and flavorful Asian-inspired dish that's perfect for weeknight dinners.

4. **Quinoa Soup:** Simmer cooked quinoa with vegetables, broth, and seasonings to create a hearty and nutritious soup that's

perfect for cold weather or when you're feeling under the weather.

5. **Quinoa Breakfast Bowl:** Serve cooked quinoa as a breakfast cereal alternative, topped with fruits, nuts, seeds, and a drizzle of honey or maple syrup for a nutritious and satisfying breakfast option.

Radishes Diet

Definition: The radishes diet involves incorporating radishes as a nutritious and versatile vegetable into meals or snacks. Radishes are low in calories, rich in fiber, vitamins (such as vitamin C and vitamin K), minerals (such as potassium and calcium), and antioxidants, making them a valuable addition to any diet.

Ingredients:

- **Radishes:** The star ingredient, rich in fiber, vitamins, minerals, and antioxidants, serves as the foundation of this diet.

- **Other Vegetables:** Pair radishes with a variety of vegetables such as carrots, cucumbers, bell peppers, or tomatoes for added flavor, texture, and nutrients.

- **Leafy Greens:** Toss radish slices with mixed greens, avocado, nuts, and a citrus vinaigrette for a refreshing and nutrient-rich salad.

- **Whole Grains:** Serve radishes alongside whole grains like quinoa, brown rice, or barley for added fiber and sustained energy.

- **Proteins:** Pair radishes with proteins like grilled chicken, tofu, chickpeas, or hard-boiled eggs to create balanced and satisfying meals.

Instructions:

1. **Radish Salad:** Combine thinly sliced radishes with other vegetables, herbs, nuts, and a balsamic vinaigrette for a refreshing and crunchy salad that's perfect for summer.

2. **Radish Slaw:** Shred radishes and cabbage, then toss with carrots, scallions, cilantro, lime juice, and a touch of honey for a crisp and tangy slaw that pairs well with grilled meats or fish.

3. **Pickled Radishes:** Slice radishes thinly and pickle them in a mixture of vinegar, water, sugar, and salt for a tangy and crunchy condiment that's perfect for tacos, sandwiches, or salads.

4. **Roasted Radishes:** Toss whole radishes with olive oil, salt, and pepper, then roast in the oven until tender and caramelized for a delicious and unexpected side dish that's perfect for roasts or grilled meats.

5. **Radish Dip:** Blend cooked radishes with Greek yogurt, garlic, lemon juice, and herbs for a creamy and flavorful dip that's perfect for serving with raw vegetables or whole grain crackers.

Raspberries Diet

Definition: The raspberries diet involves incorporating raspberries as a nutritious and flavorful fruit into meals or snacks. Raspberries are low in calories, rich in fiber, vitamins (such as vitamin C and vitamin K), minerals (such as manganese and potassium), and antioxidants, making them a delicious and nutritious addition to any diet.

Ingredients:

- **Raspberries:** The star ingredient, rich in fiber, vitamins, minerals, and antioxidants, serves as the foundation of this diet.

- **Other Fruits:** Pair raspberries with other fruits such as strawberries, blueberries, or peaches for added flavor, sweetness, and variety.

- **Greek Yogurt:** Combine raspberries with Greek yogurt for a creamy and nutritious breakfast or snack option that's rich in protein and probiotics.

- **Nuts and Seeds:** Sprinkle raspberries over nuts or seeds like almonds, walnuts, or chia seeds for added texture, healthy fats, and nutritional variety.

- **Whole Grains:** Serve raspberries alongside whole grains like oatmeal, quinoa, or whole grain toast for added fiber and sustained energy.

Instructions:

1. **Fresh Raspberries:** Enjoy ripe raspberries on their own as a refreshing and nutritious snack.

2. **Raspberry Smoothie:** Blend raspberries with other fruits, Greek yogurt, nut milk, and a scoop of protein powder for a creamy and refreshing smoothie that's packed with vitamins, minerals, and protein.

3. **Raspberry Salad:** Toss fresh raspberries with mixed greens, goat cheese, toasted nuts, and a balsamic vinaigrette for a refreshing and nutrient-rich salad that's perfect for lunch or dinner.

4. **Raspberry Chia Jam:** Cook raspberries with chia seeds, lemon juice, and a touch of honey or maple syrup until thickened for a delicious and naturally sweet jam that's perfect for spreading on toast or oatmeal.

5. **Raspberry Parfait:** Layer raspberries with Greek yogurt, granola, and a drizzle of honey or maple syrup for a

nutritious and satisfying parfait that's perfect for breakfast or dessert.

Salmon Diet

Definition: The salmon diet involves incorporating salmon as a nutritious and flavorful source of protein into meals. Salmon is rich in omega-3 fatty acids, protein, vitamins (such as vitamin D and B vitamins), minerals (such as selenium and potassium), and antioxidants, making it a valuable addition to any diet.

Ingredients:

- **Salmon:** The star ingredient, rich in omega-3 fatty acids, protein, vitamins, minerals, and antioxidants, serves as the foundation of this diet.

- **Vegetables:** Pair salmon with a variety of vegetables such as asparagus, broccoli, Brussels sprouts, or sweet potatoes for added flavor, texture, and nutrients.

- **Whole Grains:** Serve salmon alongside whole grains like quinoa, brown rice, or farro for added fiber and sustained energy.

- **Leafy Greens:** Serve salmon with mixed greens, avocado, nuts, and a citrus vinaigrette for a refreshing and nutrient-rich salad.

- **Healthy Fats:** Incorporate sources of healthy fats such as olive oil, avocado, nuts, or seeds to enhance satiety and nutrient absorption.

Instructions:

1. **Grilled Salmon:** Grill salmon fillets with a sprinkle of salt, pepper, and lemon juice until cooked through for a simple and delicious main dish that's perfect for summer.

2. **Baked Salmon:** Bake salmon fillets with a drizzle of olive oil, garlic, and herbs until flaky and tender for an easy and nutritious entree option that's perfect for weeknight dinners.

3. **Salmon Salad:** Flake cooked salmon over mixed greens, avocado, nuts, and a citrus vinaigrette for a refreshing and nutrient-rich salad that's perfect for lunch or dinner.

4. **Salmon Bowl:** Build a salmon bowl with cooked salmon as the base, then top with vegetables, whole grains, avocado, and a drizzle of tahini or soy sauce for a satisfying and customizable meal option.

5. **Salmon Tacos:** Fill corn tortillas with flaked salmon, cabbage slaw, avocado, and a squeeze of lime for a flavorful and nutritious taco option that's perfect for Taco Tuesday.

Shrimp Diet

Definition: The shrimp diet involves incorporating shrimp as a nutritious and versatile source of protein into meals. Shrimp is low in calories, rich in protein, vitamins (such as vitamin B12 and vitamin D), minerals (such as selenium and zinc), and antioxidants, making it a valuable addition to any diet.

Ingredients:

- **Shrimp:** The star ingredient, rich in protein, vitamins, minerals, and antioxidants, serves as the foundation of this diet.

- **Whole Grains:** Pair shrimp with whole grains like brown rice, quinoa, or whole grain pasta for added fiber and sustained energy.

- **Vegetables:** Serve shrimp with a variety of vegetables such as zucchini, bell peppers, tomatoes, or spinach for added flavor, texture, and nutrients.

- **Healthy Fats:** Incorporate sources of healthy fats such as olive oil, avocado, nuts, or seeds to enhance satiety and nutrient absorption.

- **Herbs and Spices:** Flavor shrimp dishes with herbs, spices, and seasonings like garlic, ginger, chili powder, or paprika to enhance taste and aroma.

Instructions:

1. **Shrimp Stir-Fry:** Stir-fry shrimp with vegetables, garlic, ginger, and soy sauce for a quick and flavorful Asian-inspired dish that's perfect for busy weeknights.

2. **Grilled Shrimp Skewers:** Thread shrimp onto skewers with vegetables like bell peppers, onions, and cherry tomatoes, then grill until cooked through for a delicious and colorful main dish that's perfect for summer barbecues.

3. **Shrimp Pasta:** Toss cooked shrimp with whole grain pasta, tomatoes, spinach, garlic, and olive oil for a light and flavorful pasta dish that's perfect for lunch or dinner.

4. **Shrimp Salad:** Serve chilled shrimp over mixed greens, avocado, nuts, and a citrus vinaigrette for a refreshing and nutrient-rich salad that's perfect for hot days.

5. **Shrimp Tacos:** Fill corn tortillas with cooked shrimp, cabbage slaw, avocado, and a squeeze of lime for a flavorful and nutritious taco option that's perfect for Taco Tuesday.

Strawberries Diet

Definition: The strawberries diet involves incorporating strawberries as a nutritious and flavorful fruit into meals or snacks. Strawberries are low in calories, rich in fiber, vitamins (such as vitamin C and vitamin K), minerals (such as manganese and potassium), and antioxidants, making them a delicious and nutritious addition to any diet.

Ingredients:

- **Strawberries:** The star ingredient, rich in fiber, vitamins, minerals, and antioxidants, serves as the foundation of this diet.

- **Other Fruits:** Pair strawberries with other fruits such as bananas, blueberries, or peaches for added flavor, sweetness, and variety.

- **Greek Yogurt:** Combine strawberries with Greek yogurt for a creamy and nutritious breakfast or snack option that's rich in protein and probiotics.

- **Nuts and Seeds:** Sprinkle chopped strawberries over nuts or seeds like almonds, walnuts, or chia seeds for added texture, healthy fats, and nutritional variety.

- **Whole Grains:** Serve strawberries alongside whole grains like oatmeal, quinoa, or whole grain toast for added fiber and sustained energy.

Instructions:

1. **Fresh Strawberries:** Enjoy ripe strawberries on their own as a refreshing and nutritious snack.

2. **Strawberry Smoothie:** Blend strawberries with other fruits, Greek yogurt, nut milk, and a scoop of protein powder for a

creamy and refreshing smoothie that's packed with vitamins, minerals, and protein.

3. **Strawberry Salad:** Toss sliced strawberries with mixed greens, goat cheese, toasted nuts, and a balsamic vinaigrette for a refreshing and nutrient-rich salad that's perfect for lunch or dinner.

4. **Strawberry Jam:** Cook strawberries with a touch of honey or maple syrup until soft, then mash or blend until smooth for a delicious and naturally sweet jam that's perfect for spreading on toast or oatmeal.

5. **Strawberry Parfait:** Layer sliced strawberries with Greek yogurt, granola, and a drizzle of honey or maple syrup for a nutritious and satisfying parfait that's perfect for breakfast or dessert.

Lentils Diet

Definition: The lentils diet involves incorporating lentils as a versatile and nutritious legume into meals to boost protein, fiber, vitamins, and minerals intake. Lentils are an excellent source of plant-based protein, making them a valuable addition to vegetarian and vegan diets.

Ingredients:

- **Lentils:** The star ingredient, rich in protein, fiber, vitamins (such as folate and vitamin B6), and minerals (such as iron and magnesium), serves as the foundation of this diet.

- **Vegetables:** Pair lentils with a variety of vegetables such as carrots, onions, tomatoes, spinach, or bell peppers for added flavor, texture, and nutrients.

- **Whole Grains:** Serve lentils alongside whole grains like brown rice, quinoa, or whole wheat couscous for added fiber and sustained energy.

- **Herbs and Spices:** Flavor lentil dishes with herbs, spices, and seasonings like garlic, cumin, coriander, or smoked paprika to enhance taste and aroma.

- **Healthy Fats:** Incorporate sources of healthy fats such as olive oil, avocado, nuts, or seeds to enhance satiety and nutrient absorption.

Instructions:

1. **Lentil Soup:** Simmer lentils with vegetables, broth, and seasonings to create a hearty and nutritious soup that's perfect for cold weather or when you're feeling under the weather.

2. **Lentil Salad:** Toss cooked lentils with mixed greens, chopped vegetables, herbs, nuts, seeds, and a vinaigrette for a

refreshing and satisfying salad that's packed with plant-based protein and fiber.

3. **Lentil Curry:** Cook lentils with coconut milk, tomatoes, onions, garlic, ginger, and curry spices for a flavorful and comforting curry dish that pairs well with rice or naan.

4. **Lentil Stew:** Combine lentils with root vegetables, tomatoes, broth, and herbs in a slow cooker or Instant Pot for a hearty and nourishing stew that's easy to prepare and perfect for meal prep.

5. **Lentil Tacos:** Fill taco shells or tortillas with seasoned lentils, lettuce, tomatoes, avocado, salsa, and a squeeze of lime for a tasty and nutritious meatless taco option that's suitable for vegetarians and vegans.

Mango Diet

Definition: The mango diet emphasizes the incorporation of mangoes as a primary source of vitamins, minerals, and antioxidants into meals or snacks. Mangoes are renowned for their high vitamin C content, as well as their fiber, vitamin A, and potassium, making them a delicious and nutritious addition to any diet.

Ingredients:

- **Mango:** The star ingredient, rich in vitamin C, vitamin A, fiber, and antioxidants, serves as the foundation of this diet.

- **Other Fruits:** Pair mango with other fruits such as berries, pineapple, or kiwi for added flavor, sweetness, and variety.

- **Greek Yogurt:** Combine mango with Greek yogurt for a creamy and nutritious breakfast or snack option that's rich in protein and probiotics.

- **Nuts and Seeds:** Sprinkle chopped mango over nuts or seeds like almonds, walnuts, or chia seeds for added texture, healthy fats, and nutritional variety.

- **Whole Grains:** Serve mango alongside whole grains like quinoa, brown rice, or whole grain toast for added fiber and sustained energy.

Instructions:

1. **Mango Smoothie:** Blend mango chunks into smoothies along with other fruits, leafy greens, Greek yogurt, nut milk, and a scoop of protein powder for a tropical and refreshing beverage that's packed with vitamins, minerals, and protein.

2. **Mango Salsa:** Dice mango and combine with chopped tomatoes, onions, cilantro, jalapeno, lime juice, and a pinch of salt for a flavorful and vibrant salsa that pairs well with grilled fish or chicken.

3. **Mango Salad:** Combine sliced mango with mixed greens, avocado, red onion, toasted nuts, and a citrus vinaigrette for

a refreshing and nutrient-rich salad that's perfect for summer.

4. **Mango Chia Pudding:** Mix pureed mango with chia seeds and almond milk, then let it sit in the fridge until thickened for a creamy and satisfying pudding that's rich in fiber, protein, and omega-3 fatty acids.

5. **Mango Sorbet:** Blend frozen mango chunks with a splash of coconut water or orange juice until smooth, then freeze until firm for a refreshing and healthy dessert option that's perfect for hot days.

Almond Butter Diet

Definition: The almond butter diet involves incorporating almond butter as a nutritious and flavorful spread into meals or snacks. Almond butter is made from ground almonds and is rich in healthy fats, protein, fiber, vitamins (such as vitamin E and vitamin B2), minerals (such as magnesium and manganese), and antioxidants, making it a valuable addition to any diet.

Ingredients:

- **Almond Butter:** The star ingredient, rich in healthy fats, protein, fiber, vitamins, minerals, and antioxidants, serves as the foundation of this diet.

- **Fruits:** Pair almond butter with fruits such as apples, bananas, or berries for a sweet and satisfying snack option that's rich in flavor and nutrients.

- **Whole Grains:** Spread almond butter on whole grain toast, crackers, or rice cakes for a nutritious and energizing snack or breakfast option.

- **Smoothies:** Add a scoop of almond butter to smoothies along with fruits, leafy greens, nut milk, and a scoop of protein powder for a creamy and nutritious beverage that's perfect for breakfast or post-workout recovery.

- **Vegetables:** Dip vegetable sticks such as carrots, celery, or bell peppers into almond butter for a crunchy and satisfying snack option that's rich in fiber and nutrients.

Instructions:

1. **Almond Butter Toast:** Spread almond butter on whole grain toast and top with sliced bananas, a sprinkle of cinnamon, and a drizzle of honey for a delicious and nutritious breakfast option.

2. **Almond Butter Smoothie Bowl:** Blend almond butter with frozen bananas, spinach, almond milk, and a scoop of protein powder until smooth, then top with granola, berries, coconut flakes, and a drizzle of almond butter for a satisfying and Instagram-worthy breakfast or snack option.

3. **Almond Butter Energy Balls:** Mix almond butter with rolled oats, honey, and a touch of vanilla extract, then roll into balls and refrigerate until firm for a convenient and nutritious snack option that's perfect for on-the-go.

4. **Almond Butter Stir-Fry Sauce:** Whisk almond butter with soy sauce, garlic, ginger, and a splash of rice vinegar until smooth, then drizzle over stir-fried vegetables, tofu, or chicken for a creamy and flavorful sauce that's perfect for Asian-inspired dishes.

5. **Almond Butter Dressing:** Blend almond butter with lemon juice, olive oil, garlic, and herbs until smooth, then drizzle over salads or roasted vegetables for a creamy and flavorful dressing option that's rich in nutrients and flavor.

Artichokes Diet

Definition: The artichokes diet involves incorporating artichokes as a nutritious and flavorful vegetable into meals. Artichokes are low in calories, rich in fiber, vitamins (such as vitamin C and vitamin K), minerals (such as potassium and magnesium), and antioxidants, making them a valuable addition to any diet.

Ingredients:

- **Artichokes:** The star ingredient, rich in fiber, vitamins, minerals, and antioxidants, serves as the foundation of this diet.

- **Dips:** Serve steamed or roasted artichokes with dips such as garlic aioli, lemon butter, or tahini for added flavor and indulgence.

- **Salads:** Add cooked artichoke hearts to salads along with mixed greens, tomatoes, cucumbers, olives, and feta cheese for a refreshing and nutrient-rich salad option.

- **Pasta:** Toss cooked artichoke hearts with whole grain pasta, cherry tomatoes, spinach, garlic, and olive oil for a light and flavorful pasta dish that's perfect for summer.

- **Pizza:** Top pizza dough with tomato sauce, mozzarella cheese, cooked artichoke hearts, roasted red peppers, and fresh basil for a delicious and gourmet pizza option.

Instructions:

1. **Steamed Artichokes:** Steam whole artichokes until tender, then serve with a side of melted butter or aioli for dipping for a simple and delicious appetizer or side dish option.

2. **Stuffed Artichokes:** Hollow out cooked artichokes and fill with a mixture of breadcrumbs, garlic, herbs, and Parmesan cheese, then bake until golden and crispy for a flavorful and indulgent appetizer or main dish option.

3. **Artichoke Dip:** Blend cooked artichoke hearts with Greek yogurt, garlic, lemon juice, and Parmesan cheese until

smooth for a creamy and flavorful dip that's perfect for serving with crackers, bread, or vegetable sticks.

4. **Artichoke and Spinach Quiche:** Mix cooked artichoke hearts with sautéed spinach, onions, eggs, milk, and cheese, then pour into a pie crust and bake until set for a delicious and hearty brunch or dinner option.

5. **Grilled Artichokes:** Halve cooked artichokes and grill until charred and tender, then drizzle with olive oil and sprinkle with salt and pepper for a smoky and flavorful side dish or appetizer option.

THE END